WE
SWIM
TO THE
SHARK

WE
SWIM
TO THE
SHARK

Overcoming fear
one fish at a time

GEORGIE
CODD

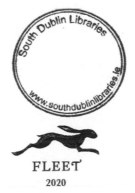

FLEET
2020

FLEET

First published in Great Britain in 2020 by Fleet

1 3 5 7 9 10 8 6 4 2

PADI excerpts published by PADI, 30151 Tomas,
Rancho Santa Margarita, CA 92688 USA.

*In order to maintain anonymity in some instances, the author has changed
the names of certain individuals, as well as identifying characteristics and details
such as physical properties, occupations and places of residence.*

A CIP catalogue record for this book
is available from the British Library.

Hardback ISBN 978-0-7088-9917-5
C format ISBN 978-0-7088-9918-2

Typeset in Bembo by M Rules
Printed and bound in Great Britain by
Clays Ltd, Elcograf S.p.A.

Papers used by Fleet are from well-managed forests
and other responsible sources.

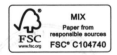

Fleet
An imprint of
Little, Brown Book Group
Carmelite House
50 Victoria Embankment
London EC4Y 0DZ

An Hachette UK Company
www.hachette.co.uk

www.littlebrown.co.uk

FOR GRANNY CODD

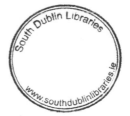

I'm up to my waist in dark water, looking back, looking forward. It's early. No one else is on this New Zealand beach apart from Alex, my travel companion and friend, who is standing by the sand dunes, wrapped snugly in a coat and scarf. She waits, a distant moral support, ready to call for help if I start to drown. The waves are calm and cold and I'm looking for shapes, which is difficult, because that's also exactly what I don't want to see. So I'm looking while trying not to look. Skimming the sea with my eyes.

I wade and wade until I have no option but to swim. I spot something ahead of me, far out in the water. A black dot rises up and then it's gone. Might have been a trick of the eye. But then – maybe I see another one. Yes. There are two.

I want to go back to the beach.

A glaring crimson line splits the sky. I'm so out of my depth I could put on stilts and still not touch the bottom. I can barely see Alex. She could be anyone, over there. And in here I am no one. A pair of legs, a pair of arms, a pair of fast-breathing lungs. In here I'm too human. And now my pair of human eyes sees that those black dots aren't dots any more. They're fins. Unmistakably. They're about 20 metres away. They're coming closer. Then they're gone.

No word could be large enough to describe the size of my panic. Fear courses through me, setting my mind to a state of hyper alertness. My reflexes hone in on every noise, every sensation, and recoil. *What's that? What's this? What's beneath me? Is it under my feet?*

I start to sing, hoping that the sound of my own voice will make this situation feel more familiar. What comes out of my mouth is not something I've ever sung before. It's tuneless. More just a rhythm. I sing, 'Please go away please go away please go away' in a falsely upbeat tone, like, no, this isn't bothering me, there aren't any sea creatures here, 'Please go away.' But, at the very furthest reaches of my brain, I can also hear myself thinking something else. A phrase I cannot say out loud.

Come here.

And then it does: a single black shape directly in front of me; a monolith rising up, leaning forward, sinking down. It's the fin of a dolphin. An adult dolphin. And it's so close. Four metres away. Three.

It is silent. Eye level. Touching distance.

And now gone. But I have no idea where.

There's a sudden spurting noise behind my head. *Pah.*

I thrash and turn. It's gone again, with nothing left to show for it. Not even a ripple.

I realise that the dolphin must be circling me. It is darting between my naked feet, the master of grey water I can't see through. When I look up more fins are approaching. This is quite a lot like a nightmare. More awful than a nightmare though: with my eyes open it gets worse. Two more fins are coming. How can this be an experience that little children dream of? Who could think that swimming with a pod of dolphins would be a fun thing to do? Why did *I* think it would be a fun thing to do? These creatures are wild. Indecipherable. Anything could happen.

Still out of my depth, and very much outnumbered, I'm

close to hyperventilating. I've got to go. I've been in for less than ten minutes but it's too long and I'm not ready. I start to swim back to shore. I need Alex to be bigger. I need to be bigger. Because right now I am tiny and I don't like it.

Some time ago, a man I met told me he'd dived with two wild dolphins. His name was Paul. As Paul and his dive buddy floated underwater, the dolphins started to mimic them, raising themselves up as if standing, hovering soundlessly opposite in the blue. Staring.

Paul's friend, James Deane – the owner of a dive shop in South London – is also suspicious of wild dolphins. When we talked about fear and the sea, that's what he told me. 'The only time I've ever been truly scared was with dolphins,' he said. That was during a dive in which he found himself surrounded by fifty of them, or more. The water was murky, he said. The dolphins had smiley faces, he said. When he saw them he thought, *They're up to something.*

As soon as my feet meet the seabed, I can breathe again. Until this moment I never realised how closely my feet and lungs worked together. I can stand and not lose my breath. I can look back out to the open water, and, with solid ground underneath me, the fins don't seem like so much of a threat. They're still sinister, yes, but they're further away now. And Alex is closer. I wave to her and a coat-wrapped arm waves back. Good old Alex. Now I can see there are other people gathering on the beach, only they're stripping down and pointing at the fins and looking enthralled, not scared.

I try to picture this scene the way they're seeing it.

Black fins good.

Black fins good.

They're coming into the water, these people – two men

and a woman – and they're so delighted to be here; to be this close to the pod.

I want to be that delighted.

A large wave looms. Two shadows are caught inside it and they're racing. The other bathers squeal with pleasure. There's a baby dolphin playing near them now. It jumps. Makes a splash.

For a second, this looks almost enjoyable. And in that moment I feel myself being pulled towards them. There's a current inside me, dragging me back. It is terrifying. And I can't seem to escape it.

Part One

We Dive

1

Big Fear

'*Dive only when feeling well, both physically and mentally.
You should be confident about the dive. Be sure the dive and
its activities are within your capabilities. Remember – diving
is supposed to be fun.*'

DIVE SAFETY PRACTICES SUMMARY,
PADI OPEN WATER MANUAL, 1999–2007

I learned to fear fish over several years, never knowing I was
taking secret lessons. According to the research I've been
doing, that's how these things can happen. At the moment
of birth we pop out phobia-free, scared only of falls and loud
noises, until life teaches us otherwise. For my mum's mum,
Granny Codd, the lesson came when she was still a baby: her
sleeping aunt (my great-great aunt) rolled on top of her in the
bed. She might have suffocated had her mother (my great-
grandmother) not heard Granny's muffled cries. Even now,
in her nineties, she still can't stand her face being covered or
touched. Not by hands. Not by fabric. Not by water.

In our earliest stages, all of us have the potential to be
Little Albert, a baby who's famous in psychological circles for

appearing, in 1920, in a short but influential film and report. When Little Albert entered the world of science, he was nine months old, had been borrowed from his mother, and was judged to be emotionally stable. Monkeys, dogs, rabbits – none of them bothered him. Not until two psychologists decided to strike steel with a hammer whenever Little Albert touched a live white rat. Like all babies, Albert didn't enjoy the loud noises. Loud noises made him cry. But that didn't stop the psychologists striking the steel – quite the opposite: they kept it up. Soon, whenever he saw anything furry, Albert would become afraid and start crying. He had been conditioned to associate furry things (rat) with horrible things (steel hit with hammer). And suddenly Albert was scared not only of rats, but of dogs and rabbits too. He even became scared of items that were barely related to rats – inanimate things like seal-skin coats and a Santa Claus mask decorated with cotton wool.

Poor Albert. Nobody seems to know what became of him – if the scientists then un-scared him, or if he spent the rest of his days tormented by furs and Christmas. We don't know if his mother gave her consent for the experiment, or if she was able to help him feel better again. We still don't know Albert's true identity.

My own phobia was different. It didn't come on that young, or that fast. Fish did not concern me for most of my childhood. Spending long days at Granny Codd's beach hut, I played in the sea every moment I could from late spring until late autumn, relishing the time I had with a grandmother who cared for me; kept me loved, fed and entertained while my mother was at work. Back then, on the rare occasions fish made an appearance, I was delighted, running back to Granny – Mum, too, at the weekends – to report all that I'd seen. I wasn't even afraid when I witnessed a classmate shriek his way out of the water near the beach hut. He'd been stung on the foot by a weever fish, and cried so loudly it made my own feet throb. Still I returned to the sea.

Perhaps my classmate's distress was some kind of foundation lesson for my later ichthyophobia. Perhaps that was the earliest seed of doubt. *Ladies and gentlemen, exhibit one.*

Exhibit two could easily have been *Jaws*, the film that launched a million sea- and shark-related fears. My cousins and I watched the movie so many times it took a bite out of my confidence – and theirs too. Even though great white sharks have never been seen near Poole, where I grew up, splashing about in the shallows. Even though Jaws is clearly made of rubber. Even though Peter Benchley, the creator of *Jaws*, spent much of his later career championing sharks as innocent creatures. 'A human being is still more likely to die of a bee sting, snake bite or, Lord knows, automobile accident than by shark attack,' he wrote in the *Guardian* in 2000. 'It's also important that we understand that the shark is not invading our territory, threatening our homes or livelihoods; we humans are the trespassers.'

According to Peter Benchley, if a shark chooses to attack us that's our fault, not the shark's. You shouldn't be in its domain. Except when the sea looks only blue and boundary-free, knowing you're in the wrong place seems near impossible.

Perhaps the shape of the shark is the clue: their bodies seem designed to indicate *DANGER. KEEP AWAY.* The dorsal fin like a sharpened arrow. The continuous snake-like motion of their tails. The purposeful black eyes. As Philippe Cousteau – son of Captain Jacques – wrote, 'The eyes [when a shark approaches head-on] are almost invisible, because of their lateral positioning, while the slit in the half-opened mouth, and the three regularly spaced fins give him the appearance of a malignant and terrifying symbol imagined by some Aztec sorcerer.'

I am, of course, aware that while all sharks are fish, not all fish are sharks. And that most fish don't even have the means to injure anyone, let alone end a human life. I know that there are many reasons *not* to be scared of this watery animal group. But similarly to poor Little Albert, those links have become entrenched. Here I am, twenty-eight years old, now living in London, more than 24 crow-flying miles from the sea, feeling more afraid of fish than ever before. And when I go back to Poole, to where I grew up – when I'm pushing Granny along the beach-side promenade in her wheelchair, listening to her stories – when she teases me about cooling off with a quick dip in the sea – I look at the waves, see each one as a fin, as *DANGER*, and I shudder.

Ridiculous though this fear might sound, apparently I'm not alone. The Barbadian singer Rihanna, I've read, feels the same way about fish. Brad Pitt, meanwhile, is scared of sharks, and Taylor Swift is creeped out by the thought of sea urchins. That's just the world of celebrity gossip.

Closer to home, I recently heard about a woman who was so phobic of fish she couldn't even sit with someone eating it. An employee of hers spilled the beans. He told me that, whenever his boss held business meetings at restaurants, no one would be allowed to order anything fishy off the menu. I wonder what she didn't like about fish. Perhaps it was the slime. Perhaps it was the eyes. Was it live fish as well as the cooked ones? Was it the smell?

I wondered what fish had done to her.

My phobia could be so much worse, I know. I could be scared of something I encounter every day. Like germs (mysophobia). Or sunlight (heliophobia). Or trees (hylophobia). I could be, like some unfortunate people, afraid of falling asleep (somniphobia). Although if I continue to have nightmares about fish appearing spontaneously, falling asleep might become the next part of the problem.

In fact, my fears have already grown bigger than pure ichthyophobia. Because, when I contemplate them properly, I can see that they are no longer exclusive to *Jaws* or weever fish. Over time, my phobia has expanded into a phobia of all sea creatures. Especially the big ones. Especially the huge ones with black eyes. Like whales. Whales are clever. They know what they're doing. The thought of meeting a whale gives me palpitations. 'The first sight of a whale in the water is terrifying,' wrote Jacques Cousteau. I can believe him.

My fear now is also not only a fear of enormous, fish-like things. It's tiny fish-like things too. The things I know are there but aren't. And emotionless things. Expressionless things. Does 'ichthyophobia' cover expressionless things?

What's the word for being a land-locked woman who dreams of great white sharks in her mother's dining room, hovering between the sideboard and the table, projecting their bloodied gums and gnashing their teeth? For someone who walks to her work at a urological clinic, comparing, with a shiver, the heights of the buildings she passes to the lengths of giant squid tentacles? Who files away pictures of bladder cancers without a moment's pause, but cannot think of coral reefs without the colour draining from her face?

These things mutate. Long after *Jaws* there was a small fish bite in Mallorca, right on my thigh, without me seeing it coming. The bite drew blood. A few years later, when I was fifteen, on a snorkelling trip to the Great Barrier Reef, I had my very first panic attack, all because fish were clustered around my face. From that point on, I knew I had a problem.

I used to love sea-swimming.

*

One day I form a plan. The plan is inspired by spiders. Eventually this plan will lead me through fear, folly and death. It will lead to a fish so terrifying I can barely conceive it exists. But all that is a long way off.

The plan is set in motion on a Friday night, while I'm trying to blot out my London life – something I try to do almost every weekend. On this particular Friday, instead of spending our free time looking for new towns to move to, or travelling back to Poole where Granny Codd sits in her nursing home (instructing us to enjoy ourselves without her in one breath; hinting at how more visits would be welcome in the next – 'The other people here are so dreary and *dull*'), my boyfriend Ted and I pick the third of our stock weekend options and ride the train to Oxford, his childhood home. We've been doing this since we first got together, five years ago, during a writing course: spending a weekend with his parents every month or two for a break. There's clean air and good company here. A happy interlude from grimy London.

On the Saturday, after a day of canal walks and reading, Ted pub-hops with his mates and I catch up with an old school friend who's living on the other side of the city. Over pizza and wine, Mandi tells me she was recently enlisted in an Oxford University trial that looked at conquering fears with cognitive behavioural therapy (CBT) – a therapy that talks through issues by linking thoughts and feelings with bodily reactions. Mandi's fear was spiders. And her fear of spiders was huge. After a general CBT introduction, she says, the researcher showed her pictures of spiders on a computer screen. These were interspersed with words, some positive, some negative. *Don't look away from these spiders, Mandi. How do they make you feel?* Mandi freaked out. She started to shake. Her heart rate rocketed. She tells me she thought she was actually going to die.

In another part of the trial, Mandi was shown a dead house spider in a sealed transparent petri dish, then asked what would happen if she was forced to hold the spider in her palm. 'I'd have to cut my hand off,' said Mandi. 'I would never feel clean again if I didn't.' I laugh when I hear this. Mandi laughs too. But she stresses she wasn't exaggerating. She says, 'I genuinely would have had to cut off my hand.' The first time she said this, during the trial, the researcher didn't laugh. Instead she talked Mandi through that feeling, helping her to think more objectively about the situation – that the spider was dead; that it was safely sealed away in plastic – and eventually Mandi was able to hold the edge of the petri dish. It was an improvement.

The last task of the day involved seeing just how near Mandi could get to a tarantula in a tank. The tank was down the end of a corridor, a fair distance away from the room they had spent their time in. Despite the distance, for a long while Mandi couldn't even enter the start of the corridor. She would take a step in, panic, then step back. Keeping behind her, patiently waiting, the researcher timed Mandi's progress with a stopwatch. After a very long while, full of retreats, hesitation, tremors and sweating, Mandi came as close as one metre away. She could not get any closer.

Throughout these tasks the researcher performed therapeutic activities to remind Mandi she was safe, to top up the rational part of her brain – the part that says spiders are mostly harmless; that you're much more of a threat to them; the kind of thing Granny Codd will say before telling you to leave the little spider in her hair. ('It's a money spider,' she says. 'Don't let me forget to buy a Lottery ticket for Saturday.') More importantly, the researcher taught Mandi exactly how panic responses work: that fear cannot grow infinitely. Our bodies cannot sustain it. Instead it reaches a high point and then plateaus. You have to stay with your panic, Mandi learned. If you run, your body thinks that's the only option it has to feel safe again. But if you stay with your fears and wait, if you watch your responses work, you'll see that your body will calm itself in time.

Mandi tells me how, a few weeks later, she went back to the Oxford researcher for a follow-up. Again she was shown pictures. *Look at this spider. How does it make you feel?* With what she had learned before still fresh in her mind, this time Mandi freaked out less. The sweats were down. The shaking was under control. She was calmer with the petri dish. And when it came to the tarantula, Mandi was able to walk straight up to it without hesitation. More. She could touch the tank.

Mandi still feels apprehensive of spiders, she tells me. But not the kind of scared that makes her think she is going to die. If she keeps up the CBT, she reckons, she might even be able to touch the spider itself one day. Her phobia's on the wane.

On my way walking back to Ted's parents' house, I make a resolution. I am going to try my own experiment. Following Mandi's example, but without a team of academic researchers, I am going to build up my resistance to fish; to take the fire out of my phobia; to use my rational brain and trick the rest of me into compliance.

Yes, I think, walking the lamp-lit pavement I've walked many times before. *And for that I'll need to find my own underwater tarantula.*

My chest tightens. With every footstep I take the idea grows. And so does the size of the fish I think about facing.

Back in London, the idea continues to gather momentum, never more so than when I'm at work. When I'm standing in the urology clinic's windowless filing room, punching holes in blood test results. When I'm rearranging boxes for our next audit. When I'm counting the minutes until I can shut down my PC. At the clinic, my purpose feels pointless. In London, too. In this set-up that I've built over the past few years. Anyone could do what I've been doing, and end up with the same result: an existence which is bland, but salaried; that only works to sustain its own continuation. I tell myself how lucky I am. I have a place to live, a person to love, and a job that pays more than the minimum wage. But it feels like something's missing.

I'd thought that, by this age, I might feel like an adult. Independent. Free. I'd thought I'd be breaking out and having adventures; earning more than small change to be hoovered up into London's bottomless money pit. Ted and I could be exploring right now. Doing all the things we're able to do before we're in a nursing home ourselves. But we aren't.

I contemplate the options. It's not enough for me to keep dipping my toes in British waters, then run out. A short snorkelling trip might test me, might get my heart rate pumping, but I know that it won't involve coming face to face with my tarantula. I want something grander, more enduring. I want to track down the biggest, scariest fish in the ocean, look into its massive eyes, and say 'I'm not afraid.'

Online, at home, I search for it: the largest; the one with the darkest mouth and heaviest look. I want eyes that stare. A tail, veering. A body that goes on and on. One contender rises above the others. Putting myself beside it in my mind, I break out into goose bumps and pull away. If I go ahead with this I'll need to learn how to get close. How to stay immersed. It dawns on me: I'll need to learn how to scuba dive. Then, once that's done, I must learn how to make myself swim with it. The biggest fish of them all.

The mighty, monstrous whale shark.

Suddenly, my next few months have meaning. They have

shape. In the midst of that shape I imagine quitting my job. Leaving London with Ted and staying out of it. Meeting Goliath. If I do all these things, I will not only deal with my phobia of fish, but perhaps use the process to tackle my other fears too. That would be good. I have loads.

Now is not the right time to think about those, however. Now is the time to focus and be practical. To make this work. Since leaving school I've scraped savings together, hoping that one day I will have somehow amassed enough cash for a house. I check the funds. I'm a long way from a half of a deposit, but if I'm careful I could have enough to leave work for a few months before I become officially poor. Investing in adventure beats bricks and a mortgage. Mum has bricks and a mortgage, and they're an endless source of complaints. Granny Codd has her own bricks too, and all they've done is given her something to lose; something to miss. Learning to dive, on the other hand, conquering this fear, is something that no one can take away from me. The bricks and the mortgage can wait.

In the evening, before Ted comes home, I look up flights. Places to go. Courses to take. With perfect synchronicity, my friend Alex calls to say she wants to go on a pals' trip to New Zealand. She asks if I'd like to come along and fulfil our nerdish ambitions to wander the land of *The Lord of the Rings*. It will cost more, but still it could fit with my plan. If I join Alex I can come back to the UK via Thailand, home of cheap diving and whale sharks – a visa will let me stay for up to thirty days.

Once Ted gets in from work, he and I talk it through. He's not enjoying his job either; is bored of writing emails for a customer service department. Since I'm quitting, he could quit too. We exchange ideas. Ted isn't fussed about New Zealand – 'Very happy for you ladies to invade Hobbiton without me' – nor is he bothered about going in on dive lessons. Instead he proposes to join me after I've found myself a whale shark. To holiday in the calm after the storm.

Together we form the rest of the plan: once I've defeated fear itself, the two of us will have a low-cost inland adventure in Chiang Mai and Bangkok. After that, back in the UK, I will move down to Bristol, a place we'd both like to live in, and volunteer on a farm so I can stay near the city rent-free. While I'm volunteering I will also look for jobs in the local area. As soon as I've found one, Ted will leave *his* job and come down to Bristol to join me. We will rent a house together – in Montpelier, maybe, or as close to Clifton as we can afford. I'll support us while Ted bags a new place to work. We will escape. We will be happy. No longer will we be renting our home off his parents as we have for the past five years; we'll be properly self-sufficient, and I will not be worried about being stuck. Or perhaps the diving will spark something else entirely. Perhaps we'll move abroad, to somewhere with clear, warm water and luscious fruit trees. Maybe I'll become the next Captain Cousteau, living a life of colourful romps. If I can learn to conquer my phobia, anything will be possible.

Everything is falling into place.

I book the flights first. Then I plot out a month's worth of travels: two weeks with Alex at the start, two weeks with Ted at the end. After more weeks of careful research, I eventually focus on the whole point of the trip, and book on to a scuba diving course in the Gulf of Thailand. The only time I've dived before was in my local swimming pool. I was eight years old and spent the ten-minute taster session pretending to be a mermaid. The pool was fish-free and child-sized. It was no more than 2 metres deep. The most dangerous thing that could have happened in there was being kicked in the head by a fellow clumsy mer-kid. But now I'm going to try scuba diving in the open water of the sea: four days of training that start in the classroom and end 18 metres down in the Gulf. And then I'm going to enter the water with a whale shark – a fish whose tail alone grows to three times the length of my entire body.

On the day I hand in my notice at work, I can barely concentrate. My line manager receives my letter, acting disappointed, and offers to keep my job open. I can go back there on my return, he says; keep my admin manager role; even take a higher salary. I thank him and turn him down. Nothing will stop me cutting my ties to London.

After I walk out of his office my exhilaration continues to grow. New purpose. New possibilities. New Zealand. It's all fine as long as I don't think about the specifics – like what happens when I'm on my own after New Zealand. Like the practicalities of learning scuba in Thailand. Like running out of money. Specifics like the monstrous whale shark itself.

Nor do I want to face the guilt I have for planning to go away. I try not to think about willingly eroding our house deposit to embark on a personal journey. Or about making myself unavailable to visit Granny Codd in the home, despite knowing how bored and jaded she's getting. While I'm trying to deal with big fish in Thailand, my mum and aunt Josie will be the only core family visitors Granny can rely on. But that will be OK. It has to be OK. Perhaps it will encourage her to socialise with her fellow OAPs.

When I start to make my plans known I receive encouragement: from colleagues and friends who understand the pull of my ambition; people who cheer me on. Ted seems as excited as I am. Perhaps it's because he knows better than most how agitated London life has made me. He must be looking forward to an end to the tears and complaints. Even

Granny, who I've never seen enter the sea – who's gathered numerous personal stories, throughout her long life on the coast, of the terrible things it can do – urges me on the telephone to get out there and have fun, to keep a journal about my time, then send it for her to read. When I see her in person, she goes one step further and asks if she can come to Thailand with me – fails to remember, as she often does these days, that her legs don't work any more; that she can't stand up without being flanked by carers. It seems mean to remind her of why she must stay put. But soon enough she forgets and is cheerful again.

Elsewhere, my constant chatter about my plan alerts me to the presence of many divers. It turns out the country is full of them – divers who know more divers, all of whom have stories about what diving has done for them. I can't get enough of these stories. I begin to collect them and keep them close, hoarding them as evidence that what I am planning has worth.

One day, a friend of a friend puts me in touch with a diving instructor called Alex – not the Alex I'm going to New Zealand with, but another (male) Alex – and he agrees to have a chat with me on the phone. This Alex tells me he's never liked swimming, particularly when he's out of his depth. But when he dives and he can see where he's going, all that ocean-related stress evaporates.

'Scuba diving isn't for everyone, definitely,' he warns. 'But there's a lot of people who think it won't be for them, and actually it is. A good mate of mine won't normally even go in the sea at *all*, but in scuba gear he's as happy as Larry. It is absolutely possible to conquer fears you have at the beginning, and just go really far with it.'

This Alex makes me think that my self-prescribed immersion could actually work. Never mind the other things he tells

me. About drowning. About death. Ignore, ignore, ignore.
Now's not the time.

Online, I come across a diving shop in South London, and
wonder if talking to anyone there will help me prepare for
my fish-seeking adventure. This shop is a specialist shop for
divers who have received, or are receiving, what is known
as 'technical' training. These divers, also called 'teccies', are
trained to go deeper than the standard dive qualification of
30 metres, and sometimes stay underwater for several hours,
breathing in specialist mixes of air: compositions like trimix,
a gas made from helium, nitrogen and oxygen that reduces
the likelihood of hallucinations, along with other deep-sea
hazards. I want to know who these people are, that can enter
the sea so confidently, leaving their land-legs behind them
for so long.

I put together a grovelling, long-winded email, begging
to visit. A short answer comes back the next morning: 'Yep
that is not a problem the door is always open if you would
like to pop in.' When I turn up during my next day off, on a
Friday afternoon, I meet the shop's owner, James Deane (the
man who doesn't trust dolphins), for the first time. His shop
is quiet – it's a weekday after all – and filled with intense-
looking scuba kit, a 1950s motorbike and multiple items
salvaged from wrecks. Bullets, portholes, a steam whistle, an
old metal helmet. James offers me a mug of tea. He tells me
about how he dives D-Day wrecks in Normandy; how last
year they found a tibia and fibula inside a sunken ship, then a
load of other bones nearby. ('We brought them together and
laid them to rest there,' he says. 'We tried to find the skull
too, but we ran out of time at the bottom before we could.')

By the time I leave, my brain is awash with tales of scuba
adventures, not to mention a fair few notes about dives going

wrong. I find myself wanting to know much more – like a bystander gripped by the sight of unfolding disaster, watching a tidal wave rearing its head before it rolls over to crush them – and James gives me permission to be his shop's writer in residence whenever I can. Granny Codd will love this, I think to myself, as I read what I've jotted down.

On my next visit, during a bustling Saturday, fear is on the agenda. I sit on a stool beneath the masks and observe what's going on, listening for anything I can hear that might help me cope with my own issues. Whenever a customer comes to refill their tanks, buy new equipment, get measured for a drysuit, or simply stop for a chat, I start by asking each of them the same question: 'Are you ever afraid in the water?'

Even among these veterans, some of whom have dived to depths of 60 metres or more – twice the maximum limit allowed in advanced recreational diving – the answer, to my surprise, is mostly yes. This is not what I expected. Shouldn't learning to dive shake off those fears of water and darkness and creatures? I consider the idea that the therapy I'm planning might leave me with more phobias than I started with.

Please no. That's not allowed.

Out of all of the customers who stop by, Paul, a crinkly-eyed man who works in telecoms, the guy who watched dolphins mimicking him and his dive buddy, is just about the most talkative diver I meet. When we speak about fear, Paul tells me he's dived with oceanic whitetips, a fast-moving, unpredictable shark with a chilling reputation for targeting castaways. They are thought to have attacked a huge number of shipwrecked sailors in the last century alone. They have been accused of killing nearly six hundred floating survivors from the torpedoed USS *Indianapolis* in 1945, for example, as well as up to eight hundred from the torpedoed RMS *Nova Scotia* in 1942. Jacques Cousteau is said to have described whitetips as the 'most dangerous of all sharks'. Yet Paul says that, on his dive, they were fine. The appearance of an ocean sunfish, however, a large but docile creature with a glove-like body and bulbous eyes, 'scared the life out of me.'

Later he describes an incident which happened to him almost 40 metres down, and which affected him for many years afterwards. During this dive both of his breathing regulators started to freeflow – letting air out of his tanks at an uncontrolled and unsustainable rate. As he tried to sip from this flow and stay breathing, seawater rushed into his mouth. Going straight up to the surface from that depth could easily have brought on the bends, an affliction caused by the body's inability to reabsorb nitrogen bubbles due to quickly rising pressure: these bubbles can block blood flow, swell organs, contort the body (i.e. bend it) and cause death. But going straight up to the surface was all Paul wanted to do. Instead he was forced by necessity to share air from his buddy's tank. Together they made a slow and careful ascent back to the boat, giving their bodies the time they needed to decompress on the way, letting all that nitrogen dissolve instead of expand.

'I've relived that a few times,' Paul tells me. But he made himself keep diving. It's like getting back into the driver's seat after a car accident, he says. 'You've got to train yourself. Put it in a box.'

Another tec diver, Raf, shows up to drop off some air tanks for filling. At first he emphatically tells me he's never been scared, and I buy it. Then he laughs. He's pulling my leg.

'I get apprehensive when it's silted out,' he says. 'When the visibility is crap.' I picture diving and not seeing a thing. Imagine what could be in there, sensing your movements when you can't sense it. Not even being able to tell when you've slipped between a gigantic pair of jaws.

Raf and James joke about someone they know who was

so afraid on a dive that he emptied his air tank while still underwater – a rarity in diving, and highly dangerous. After hyperventilating away their own supply, this person had to move in on their buddy's and quickly ascend to safety.

'Some people get spooked more than others,' says Paul.

No doubt.

Of the sixteen divers I talk to during my initial two days in the shop, only two are female. Sam is the first of these, and also the first to reply to my question without any hesitation.

'Are you ever afraid in the sea?' I ask her.

'Yeah!' she says, widening her eyes. She's afraid when she snorkels. She's afraid when she can't touch the bottom. She's afraid when she sees deep water. But still she gets in, and there's nothing she wouldn't try swimming with. Sam tells me about how she once dived with a thresher shark, a species that grows up to 6 metres long.

'It did a sweep back and circled us, three times, and each time it came past it got closer. I kept muttering to myself, *Small mouth. Small mouth.* But it was amazing. I could have walked on water when I got to the surface.' Thresher sharks rarely attack divers or swimmers. One source I read tells me that only five cases of thresher-on-human attacks have ever been documented. Even so, Sam must have felt like she'd cheated death.

That luck can quickly run out though; the dangers of the ocean rising up without a warning. James Deane shares stories of numerous friends lost at sea, including his old business partner, Bob. Bob, like James, was a technical diver, with decades of experience logged in his books. But eight years ago, on a dive in France, he signalled ascent to his buddy and never arrived at the surface. James thinks he had a heart attack on the way, but his body was never recovered.

'Depths kept drawing him deeper and deeper,' says James.

'He always said divers like him didn't live long past sixty. He disappeared two weeks after his sixtieth birthday.'

Tales of diving deaths continue. And although I've never heard them before, they feel familiar, as if a part of my brain was made to receive them.

'My friend, Chris, died on a dive,' James tells me. 'It was all bad luck. His rebreather unit [a piece of kit used to recycle the breath and make a deep dive last longer] packed up. When he bailed off that, to a back-up tank, the regulator – his mouthpiece – got somehow pulled out from his mouth. Then his back-up reg got stuck. Because he couldn't reach it to breathe he passed out underwater.'

After that comes the man who set up his gear wrong, and went in to convulsions from oxygen poisoning. Then the crew member who died while diving off a tourist boat in Egypt. 'He might have lived if the equipment had been better,' explains Raf, who watched it happen. Other accidents can only be hinted at. The memories are too grim.

Hearing these tales, just a snapshot from a growing global community, it's striking the number of people I meet who do ignore the warnings, all fully aware that death is only a lungful away. Who continue to go back down and risk their lives, sometimes being very afraid while doing so. Do they think they're special; somehow protected from mortality? Or are they just, like Paul, all squishing their fears into boxes, weighing down the lids with compressed air?

Perhaps that's a trick I'll need to learn.

James's weekend assistant, Ethan, who wears a fluff of new moustache and a black Cousteau-style polo neck, is the only one whose story bucks the trend.

'My brother loved diving,' he tells me. 'But he got bent on a training dive in Chepstow. He had a headache. The doctor said he could either do nothing and risk brain damage, or go into the decompression chamber. He's fine now, but he doesn't want to do it any more.'

James notes my expression and picks up his cup of tea. 'We talk people out of more stuff than we sell,' he says.

I ask him if he's ever thought of giving up himself, and he ponders this for a moment. 'When Chris went, I wanted to pack it in,' he tells me.

James takes another slurp of his tea, and lays it down on the counter.

'What are we doing, eh?' he says.

2

Strange Fish

'No one but you can say what calls you to scuba diving.'

INTRODUCTION,
PADI OPEN WATER MANUAL, 1999–2007

As my trip to Thailand approaches, and my remaining days in the clinic are increasingly numbered, more and more of my conversations are haunted by the prospect of scuba diving – even more than the prospect of big fish. I wonder what these whale sharks are luring me into.

When Ted and I are at home in the evenings, I fret aloud about what might happen out there.

'Do you think I'll die?' I ask him, as he sits at his computer, sorting through a batch of music downloads.

Ted doesn't stop to look up. 'Nah,' he says.

'I *might* die though,' I say.

'You'll be fine, Gogs.'

I fold my arms. 'If I did die would you miss me?'

He sighs at his screen.

'Hello?'

Ted lets his head loll and pulls off his headphones. 'Of course I'd miss you.'

'But?'

'But you're not going to die. You'll splish around, have a whale shark of a time, and then we'll go get massages and curries.'

'You think?'

He picks up his headphones, puts them back on, and pulls a face like a comedy bulldog, with a downturned mouth and droopy eyes. 'Yep, yep, yep, yep, yep.'

Meeting with a couple of friends for a Sunday in the countryside, I discuss my upcoming travel plans by the fire in their living room. Outside, leaf-stripped oak branches hang with pellets of ice. Thailand could not be so far away, nor feel so close.

'Scuba diving is *mental*,' says my friend MC with a grimacing enthusiasm. 'There are *so* many things to go wrong. You could get *lost*, be swept away by the *tides*, not be able to see what's *coming*, run out of *air* . . .

'I mean,' he continues, 'I think about going diving and I imagine all the water streaming out of the seabed, and me just tumbling on to the rocks. At the surface, looking down, that's what I think about: falling. Even the thought of the air bubbles freaks me out.'

MC's cousin, Beth, agrees. 'I hate the idea of not being able to escape,' she says. 'You can't just jump out, can you, or you'll get the bends.' Beth tells me she did the Open Water course – the course I'm about to do – with her husband a few years before. 'I hated it,' she says. 'That bit where they make you take off your mask underwater is the worst. You can't see, you have to find it, put it back on and clear all the water out of it with your nose. I cheated. My instructor shouldn't have passed me but he did.'

A few days later, at my request, Harry – MC's father – sends a message to me outlining the full story of his own first dive in the sea. 'I was really surprised,' he writes. 'We were in the Great Barrier Reef, up near Cape Tribulation, and out of sight of land, and I was very much looking forward to it. Our instructors had told us what to do and what to expect, so I put the gear on and jumped into the water. As soon as I did I couldn't breathe smoothly or calmly, and I had all this heavy kit pulling me down; water was coming into my mouth.

'I was in there five or ten minutes at the surface and I was terrified – we were constantly drifting, and the boat seemed to be much farther away every time I came back up – but the instructor said he would accompany me down to 10 metres to see the reef. He said it wasn't deep but it felt like a fucking long way to me. It was very difficult to suppress the feeling of panic, and not shoot right back up to the surface. But if I had shot back to the surface I'd have been in trouble.'

Scuba diving is clearly a risky activity, especially when, like Harry, or the man who inhaled his whole tank full of air, the diver starts to panic in the water. Depending on the diver, there are all sorts of things which might trigger that panic. There's the feeling of constriction from the wetsuit, which tightens the deeper you get, a sensation that, for some, is like strangulation. There's the sense of claustrophobia sometimes caused by the mask, which clings around the eyes, restricting the vision like blinkers. Some people feel claustrophobic just from being in the water, or can't stand the sensation of it washing over their face – like Granny Codd. And don't forget the panic that can be triggered by fear of darkness. It is awfully dark in certain stretches of the sea.

Panic from these things, or anything else that's troubling me, and a speedy surface from the depths could burst my eardrums, rupture my lungs or bring on a case of the bends.

Alternatively, if I find myself alone, snagged in netting or seaweed, unable to calm down enough to work my way out, I could just huff up my air supply and suffocate. Or lose my apparatus and simply drown.

I'm trying to take Granny's approach to all this new unpleasantness – the approach she's used for as long as I can remember, for scraped knees, splinters and more. This approach provokes her to ask, if you've stubbed your toe for instance, whether you'd like her to take away that pain by stamping on the toes of your opposite foot. 'You won't notice the pain in the first one after that,' she will say with a smile.

Her approach works in this context, up to a point: the more I hear these kinds of diving stories, the less space I have to ruminate on fish. That can only be a positive.

Except, what I learn about whale sharks doesn't make me any less nervous. The whale shark is a formidable creature, with the power to do huge damage with its mighty bulk and powerful oesophagus. In adulthood it weighs over 20 tonnes. As my trusty Scholastic shark book puts it, that's 'heavier than a school bus full of passengers' or 'more than three male African elephants'. That's by no means the only impressive statistic. Their mouths are, on average, 1.5 metres wide. They filter through 6800 litres of water an hour. When fully grown they have zero natural predators.

There's a lot that I still don't know about whale sharks, however – despite the nerve-wracked reading I've been doing. Such as whether or not one would swallow a human whole. I want to believe that it wouldn't, but for a fish that sucks in that much water per hour it must be possible. Recently a friend let me know that only one person has ever been killed by a whale shark, and that was because they swam inside the whale shark's mouth for a dare. In doing so, said my friend, this human killed both himself and the fish. So far I've found no evidence to back this story up. Instead, as I dip into the internet to look at whale shark attack videos – the latest on my recently closed tabs, published by the *Daily Star*, 'Shark "EATS fisherman" then spits out camera in HORROR GoPro clip', not only contains the wrong shark but also no human injury – I come across an article that's both legitimate and alarming. The report is posted on the Divers Alert Network (DAN), a respected scuba diving safety organisation established more than thirty years ago.

Title: 'Diver was virtually swallowed by whale shark'.

Subtitle: 'A clearly annoyed whale shark appeared to attempt to swallow a diver. Uncharacteristic behaviour by a known gentle giant.'

The article discusses how a woman accidentally hit a whale shark on entering the water to dive with a group. Following this, the largest whale shark present began 'swimming directly at divers with its mouth wide open . . . [Multiple] divers were able to swim out of its path.' Some forty minutes later, still in the water and trying to take a photograph, the female diver recalls being 'hit hard by the whale shark,' then 'sucked into the mouth of the whale shark, head first, and half swallowed up to her thighs.' She was soon ejected back into the water with only a 'minor abrasion' to her hand. But despite the fact she survived mostly unharmed, I find myself unable to stay optimistic. The shark's behaviour seems to me like a warning: a massive fish attempting to do damage. Did it intend to swallow too, or did its gag reflex kick in? I'm determined to track down someone who knows and find out.

In the meantime, this story reads as an exercise in the obvious unpredictability of wild animals. And also as a lesson in how not to swim with a whale shark. A commentary beneath the report warns other divers to 'always be aware

of the potential risk when diving around marine animals ...
regardless of preconceived notions of danger or safety'; to
'respect their space', and to look 'before entering the water.'
I will do all of these things. If a whale shark starts to tail me
it can have as much space as it likes. That's if I can get away
fast enough. Though if the next evidence I find is anything
to go by, escaping could prove difficult.

This comes via a video entitled 'Whale shark attacks
diver'. It was uploaded to YouTube by someone called
'72Herminator' in late 2012, and, by the time I watch it (the
first time of many), it has attracted well over one million
views. In 'Whale shark attacks diver' we are in deep water, a
shiver of adult whale sharks swimming above us. I look on,
gripping the sides of my chair, as one splits from the rest of
the shoal, and approaches the diver filming. The shark seems
to have picked this diver especially. It charges at the camera,
its vast mouth opening and closing. Internal folds of skin flap
in the current, shredded like torn rags. It looks as though the
cameraperson is trying to swim back from the whale shark
as fast as they possibly can, but whoever it is does not give us
a commentary: underwater, surrounded by scuba gear, they
do not speak or shout. Nor can they get away.

That could be me, I think.

After a minute of tense chasing, the shark changes tack and
makes for another scuba diver instead. The scale of the shark
when filmed beside this person is spine-chilling. So too is
the way it relentlessly sticks to the end of the diver's fins, following their every move. As a silent tussle plays out between
them, there is no sense of up or down, just the endless blue
of an abyss. It looks like the shark is pushing his foe to the
depths, subjecting him to dangerous pressures. Vast clouds of
bubbles pour from the victim's respirator – a sign of panic,
much like his flapping hands. As these bubbles obscure the

camera's view, anything could be happening behind them. When they clear the shark is still pushing him on.

At the end of this four-minute video, orange text zooms from the front of the screen to the back, like the opening credits of *Star Wars*. 'It looked scary ...' this text says, 'But the whale shark was only playing or interested in the bubbles!!!' I have no idea how the filmmaker reached this conclusion. Can anyone claim to know what a whale shark is thinking? Surely losing control underwater is not something to be made light of with bright font and perky exclamation marks. An adversary like that could push you down to depths of almost 2000 metres. Before you got anywhere near that far, your eardrums would implode, your nerves and vessels would stretch and compress, you would pass out, your sinuses would collapse, your soft tissues would crush into a pulp. When whale shark picks on diver, it's all too clear who's likely to come out on top.

And yet, even though I know this could be me – my own sinuses flattened – my own breath inverted – I also feel I can't call off my quest. I've told everyone that it's time to face something that's bigger than me. Bigger than anything else I've known.

I've backed myself into a corner. I have no one to blame but myself.

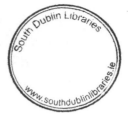

3

The Gulf

'With that first underwater breath, the door opens to a
different world. Not a world apart, but different nonetheless.
Go through that door. Your life will never be the same again.'

INTRODUCTION,
PADI OPEN WATER MANUAL, 1999–2007

I was relieved to be out of the city at first. Relieved to be
out of all cities, full stop. But too quickly that feeling,
my relief, went away. It's now only been seven hours since
Bangkok and, as the tourist ferry skims towards Koh Tao,
all I'm feeling is shit-scared. Three days ago I left Alex and
New Zealand; the hobbits and elves and frosted peaks. Five
days ago I sprinted from wild dolphins. A fortnight ago I said
goodbye to Ted, to my mum and to Granny Codd. I took
my last shift at the clinic.

I may have done a load of research since I made my decision
to come here. But still I don't feel ready for what's ahead. I
think about everything I can't see at this moment, invisible
but near. Two lidless eyes. Forty feet of night-black skin. A
mouth so wide it could swallow me into oblivion.

I think about the many other creatures suspended underneath this boat, veiled by the waters of the Gulf of Thailand. These ebbs and swells hide some 360 species of fish. Rays, barracudas, jellyfish, eels, cucumbers, slugs, crustaceans and urchins; creatures moving slowly across rock and sand. With fins. With eyes. With teeth.

I can't see them. Of course I can't see them. There are several layers of steel and wood and whatever else between us. But I know they're there. Blank faces, venomous spines. Squid, octopi, porpoises. Those creepy, shifty dolphins. And somewhere, swimming, immense, in the dark, the reason I'm here, about to learn how to dive.

Right now, my ichthyophobia has never felt more rational. I think of the fish that are found in the Gulf of Thailand.

- *Titan triggerfish*. A large, thick-lipped predator with big teeth that will aggressively defend the conical zone above its nest. Their attacks can cause serious injury.
- *Bull sharks*. A species which grows up to 3.5 metres long – territorial and aggressive. One of the most dangerous sharks in the world.
- *Lionfish*. A banded fish with venomous spines. Touching these can cause a range of reactions in humans, from vomiting and dizziness to paralysis and death.
- *Giant morays*. A carnivorous eel that grows to around 3 metres in length and hides in coral reefs. Has been documented attacking sharks as well as human beings.
- *Box jellyfish*. One of the most poisonous underwater species. Brushing past its tentacles can be extremely painful, if not fatal.

These are not the only things making me anxious. In his emails, Robert, my dive school contact, promised I'd see a friendly face as soon as I disembarked from the tourist boat. When I disembark, however, I see no friendly faces. The clump of travellers who sailed with me is dispersing, scattering between the island's beach resorts and jungle hotels. There is an age of waiting on the boardwalk. The sun sets. Then it's just me and an Englishman, making distracted efforts at conversation. He's not heading where I'm heading, and, yes, here comes his ride.

'Hope they get you soon,' he says, and he's slinging his holdall into the back of a truck.

Maybe my face looks as if this whole episode isn't bothering me. That's what I'm instructing it do. Come on, face. Behave. But the truth is I am bothered, very much. This was not part of my plan. It is night-time. The pier is deserted. My backpack is heavy. Even the last of the taxi drivers has given up waiting, after touting, unrewarded, for twenty minutes.

'You want hotel? Good price. Good price.'

'Come on, lady.'

'No? Then you sleep here.'

So I am on my own. It's dark. I'm in Thailand.

It is as if the island wants me to go home already. Give up this diving nonsense. But I'm supposed to be on a mission, and it has only just begun.

I wonder if I can walk to the dive school. It seems like madness to leave the well-lit pier. Perhaps, if I knew the way ... but then I would be a lone female, carrying hefty luggage along a series of dark and unknown paths. On New Year's Day, just a few months back, a twenty-nine-year-old Frenchman was found hanged in a bungalow near here. Though officially classed as a suicide, it's been reported that, when the Frenchman was discovered, his hands were tied behind his back, the implication being that someone else manoeuvred him into the noose. Not long before that, two

British twenty-somethings were bludgeoned to death on a nearby beach. The Burmese bar-working migrants that have been arrested for the murders are probably, reporters are saying, just a couple of handy scapegoats. And as if that wasn't enough, a little over a year ago, a young Englishman's body was found floating off the coastline. His parents are convinced he was murdered too. All of which means that at least one killer could still be walking free on this island. And that things have been happening nearby that shouldn't be happening. 'Death Island,' the tabloids are calling it.

I can't dwell on thoughts like this. It is time to try being resourceful. I get to my feet and rush around in a random series of directions. I stick to the light, keep my radius short. After a few minutes I come across a middle-aged Italian couple, wandering in a romantic fug by the harbour. I explain the situation. I'm a solo traveller; a budding diver; I'm stranded. They say they want to help but that they can't. 'Really sorry. Wish we could.' *Why* can't they help? I don't know and they're too loved-up to explain, too busy enjoying their walk to concern themselves with a panicking stranger. I keep rushing, continuing my search.

Soon I see a beacon of hope in the form of a booth labelled 'Tourist Information'. For some time I do my best to catch the eye of the man behind the glass. All the while he furiously ignores me. Instead of raising his head, he continues to scour the screen of his mobile phone. When I manage to enter his eye-line he subtly moves away, altering the boundaries. He's like some kind of anemone, the kind you'll never see fully up close because as soon as you try for a glimpse it hides away. I knock on the window. There's no response. I check my phrasebook and try, '*Sà wàt dee kâ.*'

Nothing.

'Hello?'

Not even a twitch.

'Excuse me? Can you help me?'

A female colleague of his pops her head around the corner, disturbed by the noise I've been making. She calls to him. Forces him to look at me.

He lowers his phone. 'Yes?'

'I'm sorry. Someone from my dive school was supposed to pick me up but they aren't here. Is there any way you could call them? I don't have their number.'

He shakes his head.

'Please. I don't know how to get there.'

'Take taxi,' he says.

'I don't have any cash. And the taxis have gone.'

He shakes his head again and returns to his text conversation. He clearly thinks this is not his problem. And it's a reasonable thought. I'm an idiot. Under-prepared. Dumb tourist.

'Aren't you tourist information?' I say. 'Hello? Hello?'

Koh Tao, the island on which I am currently stranded, is one of the world's most popular spots for travellers learning to scuba dive. I hear that, in the daylight, it is beautiful, that the water is both temperate and clear, and that – perhaps the biggest attraction for most – going on dives off this coastline is particularly cheap.

There are more than twenty-five dive shops on the island, all capitalising on the influx of scuba enthusiasts. For a lot of people there would be some relief in those numbers – the thousands who come here every year and apparently leave without injury (a volume of wannabe students second only to those at the Great Barrier Reef in Queensland, so I hear). But as I stand at this desk, deliberating, these are not the figures in my mind. I am thinking about how, in 2010, an Irish instructor was lost on a dive here at an underwater volcano, never to be found again. In 2013, a young father drowned on a holiday scuba trip. In 2014, a Norwegian diver was fatally injured by the propellers of a boat. And that's just what was reported in the English-speaking press.

It strikes me then: perhaps I should have looked into these incidents before coming. Perhaps I should take the dark thoughts in my head and do something positive with them. Like turn around and get back on the ferry.

I hold the counter in front of me and consider it.

In the end, it's the woman at the tourist office who gives me the help I need, though she looks even less impressed at having to do so than her colleague. He reverts to scowling at his mobile phone, while she passes me the receiver of their landline. I hear a man's voice. Gravelly. Robert, is it? No, it's not Robert. It's someone who's never heard my name before.

'Georgie Codd,' I repeat. 'Like the fish, with an extra "d". Someone was meant to come and pick me up from the pier.'

'Uh?'

'I emailed about a week ago to confirm. Don't you have a reservations book or something? Is Robert there?'

'Robert not here. No.'

'I'm supposed to start my diving lessons tomorrow. I've been waiting here for more than half an hour. Robert said someone would come to the pier and get me.'

'OK. OK. No problem. We send someone. Five minutes.'

Fifteen minutes later I'm clinging to the rear of an open truck as it zips north down the sandy road, scudding over every pothole it finds.

My guidebook told me Koh Tao was a 'jungle-topped cutie ... the busy vibe of Samui mixed with the laid-back nature of Pha-Ngan.' I have never been to Samui or Pha-Ngan, so that sentence means nothing to me. What I see on this bone-jangling ride through the dark are acres of palm tree forests dotted with starkly lit Seven Elevens, bars, bars, bars, teens, tourists and countless signs for diving courses with PADI (the Professional Association of Diving Instructors).

We soon reach our destination, where luckily there's something else to distract me: after I've checked in, a motorbike arrives for the last leg of my journey, and I find myself riding in a basket attached to the back. Riding in a basket behind a motorbike feels about as precarious as the rest of this seemingly endless day, except, for the first time, in a good way – mostly because there's a high chance of having somewhere to sleep when it's over. At last we pull up at an out-of-town hostel. It's a bit of a shack, the dorms are mixed, the loos and sinks are mere inches away from the head of my bed, but, given the rate is £4 a night, I feel foolish to have expected anything more.

Despite it now being past 9 p.m., my fellow dormers have chosen the hostel over bar-hopping tonight. After dumping my bags and splashing my face, I join them at a stone picnic table under a tree full of shrieking crickets, and piece together the lie of the land. There is a twenty-four-year-old trader, the son of American art dealers, whose specialised conversation technique involves reciting to everyone present what he saw them do today. Whenever anyone tells him he is mistaken, he argues. 'You did,' he'll insist. 'I saw you. You were eating a cheese and cream pancake, remember?' There is a tanned Finnish girl in hot pants who attracts keen male attention every time she moves. There is a short German guy in his late teens who is so high he can barely talk. There is a Peruvian boy who crashed his rental scooter and is now being forced to pay $4000 in fees by the businessman who hired it to him. From time to time, there is also a young Thai woman who dances, quite literally, in and out of the area next to the dorm rooms. Only one person here is older than I am – a thirty-three-year-old man from New Zealand. He's the most compelling talker by a long shot. A red-necked dairy farmer, he and his brother were raised by ultra-religious foster parents. Not long ago these foster parents kicked him out, and his brother committed suicide. That's when he came here to sit on a stone picnic bench and drink beer.

Only two other people around the table are also on this island for the diving. One of them is Kevin, a Scottish lad with a laugh like a scream, who has been in the hostel for two months already. He is aiming to earn his stripes as a fully fledged divemaster, and clearly considers himself king of this castle. Kevin's conversational style involves naming every animal and person that passes – 'That's Ham the dog' – 'That's Kitler the cat' – 'That's Baby the prostitute' – while reclining on top of the table, his crotch on prominent display. The other diver present is a shy-seeming American called Sarah. I leave it a while, just sit and observe, until the chance arises to ask them both if they've dived with any whale sharks. Neither of them has. Not yet.

'But they are about,' Kevin decrees. 'So it's probably only a matter of time.'

Did you hear that?

I heard that.

They *are* about, those whale sharks.

It's only a matter of time.

Thankfully, my first day on Koh Tao has nothing to do with fleeing threatening whale sharks. It barely contains any fish, apart from the small ones which join me in the shallows. Being able to see their tiny shapes through the crystalline waters doesn't trigger my usual panic responses. As long as I can see them, as long as I'm in my depth, I know I can run away in the right direction.

After firing off some desperate emails to Ted from an internet cafe – *I'm alive, I've arrived, I miss you, miss me?* – and sending a note for Granny via Mum – *DRINK MORE WATER, LADY. EAT YOUR GREENS* – that afternoon I meet my PADI dive instructor, Terry, a shaven-headed, pot-bellied Brit who wears the smell of cigarettes so thickly I suspect it will stay with him underwater. The dive school he works for hosts courses all year round. This week I am his only student and Terry's boredom is palpable. He must have taught this so many times before.

On a sweaty plastic chair in an overheated room, I fill out reams of paperwork. When I tick yes to the question about having, or having had, asthma (I grew out of it in childhood), my instructor rolls his eyes. Now, he says, I need to visit the local doctor, pay for a check-up and ask him to stamp a letter saying I'm fit enough for the course. Without it this adventure can go no further.

I sprint down the road to the nearest clinic and, still panting, puff into a well-used peak flow meter. After handing over a few baht notes, I get my stamp and sprint back to the classroom. I am now allowed to watch a two-hour, plodding introduction to the course. The film is dense with superlatives. *Best thing you'll ever do; your life will never be the same; discover new worlds.* Fear doesn't feature, but that's hardly surprising: PADI, the company that has created it – also known as the world's largest diver training organisation – has countless supplementary courses that it is urging its students to take. The last thing it wants to do is put anyone off. If I am able to complete this Open Water course, I can empty the dregs of my savings on any one of its innumerable bonus training programmes, including Advanced Open Water, Rescue Diver, Cavern Diver, Boat Diver, Altitude Diver, Sidemount Diver, Underwater Naturalist, Underwater Navigator, Underwater

Videographer – even Ice Diver. 'Flash your PADI Ice Diver certification card to get instant respect', says the PADI website. They make it sound so easy.

My second day of training is more involved. Having read the requisite chapters of the dog-eared book I've been loaned, I spend the morning watching more PSHE-style DVDs, then completing a series of photocopied quizzes. Terry yawns, sardonically mocking PADI, as he points out the book's relentless marketing, with lines encouraging me to buy branded equipment that I will apparently never need as an amateur. A thermometer. A knife. Even an electronic recreational dive planner. ('A must for all divers. Quick. Easy. Accurate.')

Soon I am introduced to the main essentials of scuba. The first surprise is that successful diving doesn't require much exertion. This would explain my instructor's shapely belly. A skilled diver should be able to adjust her buoyancy until she feels weightless, and glide through the water with just a flick of her fins. The second, more crucial, thing I learn: a diver must never, in any circumstances, hold her breath. If a breath is held, changes in pressure can mean lungs are squeezed or damaged. It's slow and steady breathing all the way.

As Terry talks me through the depths of pressure charts, I discover that diving just 10 metres down will double the normal pressure we humans experience at the surface. At the same time, our lungs' air volume is halved. I answer multiple choice questions on regulators and BCDs, otherwise known as buoyancy compensator devices – clunky vests that a diver can inflate or deflate underwater. This breakthrough piece of equipment was originally developed in the fifties and sixties, and is now a major part of most scuba kits.

After lunch it's time to get into the pool, next to which several gap-year travellers are drinking pints of Singha and sunning themselves. Some look on as I prove to Terry I can swim 200 metres, then tread water for ten long minutes without drowning. Terry seizes the opportunity to smoke, letting his fag dangle out of his mouth, dropping ash to the floor. Then it's time to meet the equipment first-hand. I clamber out of the pool, stomping my wet feet over burning tiles, and set up a heavy selection of gear. BCD, air tank, regulators and hoses, all are connected under Terry's watchful eye. I test the air and gauges, then inelegantly wrestle the whole thing on. The force of this apparatus on my shoulders makes me stoop and sway. And it's not the only heavy thing I must carry. Around my middle I also wear a weight belt, an extra measure to help me sink. For a moment I think about being made to sink, and quickly realise that brooding on this is going to be counter-productive. On go the mask and snorkel. Fins complete the look. Now I'm supposed to do my pre-dive check. I stall. I stare at Terry.

'Bruce Willis Ruins All Films,' he says.

Not *Sixth Sense*, though, I want to counter. Oh, and *Sin City*. Great film that.

Terry pauses expectantly, waiting for a dive-related response.

B.W.R.A.F. *B.W.R.A.F.* Even with the mnemonic reminder I'm struggling. Bruce is BCD. Willis is weights. Ruins is . . . Ruins is . . .

'Releases,' says Terry.

'Ah,' I say, as if that rang a bell. 'Of course.' I check my buckles and Velcro band. 'Yep,' I say. 'Checked releases.'

Terry cocks his head. 'And?'

'And . . .' I close my eyes. 'Sorry,' I say. 'It's at the tip of my tongue.'

'You need to check mine too,' he says. 'Communicate with your buddy.'

After 'All' for air, and 'Films' for final check, I shuffle back towards the pool like a hunchbacked, washed-up penguin. There's more to remember at this point too, but almost everything I've been quizzed on today has already leaked from my mind. I have to be prompted to inflate my BCD before I slide into the pool, to put the regulator in my mouth, to cover my belt with one hand and press my swimming mask to my face with the other. Then it's a shuffle off the edge and into the water with a graceless splash.

For a moment, I'm immersed. Then I pop back to the surface and bob, fully inflated, keeping my regulator in my mouth until Terry, also kitted up, drops into the water beside me. I remove the mouthpiece under instruction, and let it float face down in the pool. It looks like I've grown a tentacle. As we prepare to begin my first descent – playing with the BCD, swapping from regs to snorkel and back – I notice that another traveller has arrived among the lounging pool-side audience: the twenty-four-year old son of art dealers, David; the guy in my dorm who spends most of his time here observing other people's holidays. I say hello, and ask him if he's also going to learn diving while he's on Koh Tao. He tells me he doesn't want to. He tells me I 'look retarded'. Anyway, he says, he could pretty much do a whole fifty-minute dive just by holding his breath. Who needs all that stupid equipment? I am suddenly eager to leave the surface-dwelling world behind me. If only I could remember what the next mnemonic stands for.

Eventually we do escape humanity, or as best we can given the circumstances, as we enter the fishless domain of the chlorinated pool. It can't be much more than 3 metres deep. When I reach the bottom I catch the tips of my fins on the tiles and send myself bending awkwardly forward. I struggle to right myself for a moment, telling myself to breathe and not panic. When finally I stop flailing, Terry and I swap signals – thumb and forefinger together for *OK*, never thumbs up, which means *ascend*. (Unless we do need to ascend, that is.) Then it's time to start ticking things off the practical test. Terry shows me what to do, asks me to copy, and either slow-motion applauds or signals for me to try again. All the while my breathing is amplified, heavy and long in my ears, like some kind of end-of-life respirator, or the sound of a slasher-film murderer as he peers through a bedroom window.

From time to time, noises of splashes above also catch my attention. Lithe swimmers are floating just over our heads, refreshing themselves in the heat. Beneath them we lurk like oversized toads, performing task after task: purging air, clearing masks, removing them and swimming without, removing all our other gear and putting it back on. Apart from a few errors, I manage to keep up, but the number of things to absorb is making me increasingly nervous. It's like having your first driving lesson the day before your test, in a place where air and gravity play tricks on your wheels *and* the road. I can hardly believe that tomorrow I will be trying all this in the Gulf of Thailand, surrounded by various hordes of my scaly nemeses.

James Deane, the man who owns the dive shop in South London, once told me that, 'The trouble is, diving these days is not very dangerous.' He was only half kidding. Of course it can be dangerous. I've heard enough real-life horrors from him and his customers to make that very clear. What James really misses, he elaborated, is the sense of exploration. I sense that he yearns for the pioneering age of Jacques Cousteau, with his makeshift scuba kit; his harpoon-it-and-see bravado.

When diving first attracted widespread attention with the release of Cousteau's *The Silent World* in the fifties, anything was possible underwater. See a scary shark: kill it. Want to survey a reef fast: blow it up. Never dived before: grab the nearest air tank and head on down. Cousteau and his team of 'menfish' were lords of the sea, free to roam and try whatever they liked. The risks were all part of the game. Now recreational diving places safety first and foremost.

The remnants of Cousteau's attitude still linger, however, if James Deane and his customers are anything to go by. Each time I visited his shop I met a generation of older male divers, some out to find wrecks and treasures, others aiming to discover virgin sites in vast cave networks. A lot of these men fit a similar mould. Their compulsion to act boyishly came out in boasts and anecdotes. A dark and prankish humour.

Paul, for example, told me how he likes to shoot dogfish at his mates – coiling them into his hands, turning them upside-down and freeing them – or firing them off – seeing them hurtle forward to escape. James described how he had latched on to a sea turtle, riding it like a diver propulsion vehicle. Both men laughed about putting hermit crabs on other people's heads and watching the subsequent hysteria.

I need no extra reason to panic on the day of my first open water dive in Koh Tao, and thankfully Instructor Terry doesn't seem to be in the mood to play any tricks. I think he's just keen to get on with it, so he can head back to the bar. Our relationship isn't so much mentor and student, as dive-enabler and annoyance. I'm big, I'm uncoordinated, I'm scared of fish and I'm not signing up for more courses with him after I've done this one. There's no point trying to charm me. Representing the Korean section of the dive school, on the other hand, our more attractive counterparts – a gorgeous young woman called Mina, and her handsome older instructor, Matt – have spent twice the time that we have on their pool-work, perfecting every technique, buying each other drinks, learning the basics and then some. This afternoon the four of us will dive at the same time, and I'm under no illusion as to which of us students will have the better experience.

Last night I tried to relax in preparation for this first dive in open water. On my instructor's advice, I booked an hour with his favourite local masseuse, a Thai woman named Mango. 'Hands like Harry Potter,' Terry had said. When the time came, my massage proved to be more like a rollercoaster at Harry Potter World than the blissful, quiet encounter I'd envisaged. My body was the cart and Mango was riding. For an hour, I found myself stretched into a sequence of outrageous positions. Every time my bones clicked, limber Mango cooed my name. At one point, when only my chest and hands were in contact with the mattress, a German couple passing the window gasped so loudly I managed to hear them over Mango's noisiest '*Georgina*'.

'Are you all right?' they called. Afterwards I felt like I'd spent a week under the Whomping Willow.

As I lay in my bed recovering, the human world offered other ways to take my mind off diving. At about two o'clock in the morning, two Canadian hostelers decided to share a prostitute in my dorm.

CANADIAN NUMBER ONE: This way, this way. It's fine. Yeah.

PROSTITUTE: There girls in here?

CANADIAN NUMBER ONE: No. No girls. Come on. This is fine. Nobody minds.

AUTHOR: I do. I mind.

PROSTITUTE: A girl!

CANADIAN NUMBER TWO: No. No girls. No one minds.

AUTHOR: [louder] I mind.

CANADIAN NUMBER ONE: [stopping at the bed next to mine] Here will be good.

AUTHOR: Here is NOT good.

CANADIAN NUMBER ONE: Let's do it in here.

AUTHOR: Don't do it in here.

CANADIAN NUMBER ONE: Shut up. I want to fuck, OK? We're fucking in here.

AUTHOR: No, you're not.

CANADIAN NUMBER TWO: Be quiet. I paid 500 baht for this good time. You're not going to ruin it for us.

AUTHOR: Do it somewhere else.

CANADIAN NUMBER ONE: [undoing his trousers] Imagine it's like background music or something. Peaceful background music.

CANADIAN NUMBER TWO: Ha ha.

CANADIAN NUMBER ONE: It's like – it's like – what's that song?

AUTHOR: You cannot fuck next to my bed. I won't let you.

CANADIAN NUMBER TWO: We'll fuck behind your bed, then. In the bathroom.

AUTHOR: NO. Not in this room.

CANADIAN NUMBER ONE: Beethoven! Mozart! It's like – imagine it's like Beethoven's Ninth – Fifth – it'll be like listening to Beethoven's Fifth Symphony! Ha ha!

DAVID, TWENTY-FOUR-YEAR OLD SON OF ART DEALERS: [suddenly awake] Ha ha.

AUTHOR: [increasingly desperate]: If you start having sex in this room, I will kick you in the head.

CANADIAN NUMBER ONE: Go on. Kick me. Ha. I'd like that.

CANADIAN NUMBER TWO: You're not helping, dude.

PROSTITUTE: We go different place.

CANADIAN NUMBER ONE: NO. There is no
   different place.

On and on and on it went, until the Canadians finally left
for another dorm and shared the woman there.

Now at the dive school I'm gathering kit, helping load it on
to a truck. Before we go I visit the toilet, again and again,
too many times to count. My bowels and bladder are taps I
can't turn off. Then we're heading to the sea. We're heading
to where the wild fish live. The dolphins, the eels, the sharks.
Terry tells me we're going to do two dives of roughly forty
minutes apiece, the first in 8 metres of water, the second
down to 12. I nod, barely taking it in. Twelve metres must
be too shallow for a whale shark, I reason. At least I hope it
is. I'm not ready for that yet. I need to build myself up. Terry
lights his next cigarette, and asks if I'm all right. I tell him I
don't know.

   'You'll be fine,' he says. 'Just follow what I'm doing.'

   But I'm thinking about what happened when I went to the
Great Barrier Reef. How, as soon as I entered the water with
my snorkel, all the fish honed in on me. How, in Mallorca,
that biting thing went straight for my leg.

   We board the boat – Terry and I, plus the tight Korean
twosome – and set off across the picture-book sea. The boiling sun catches our spray as we travel, transforming it into
rainbows. Today, the scenery of Koh Tao is that of a typical
tropical paradise: leaning palm trees, dense green forest, all
this sparkling blue.

   We approach our first stop and Terry supervises my gear
check, helps me into the BCD, watches me do up my buckles.
The engines cut out. For a moment I think we have broken

down, but in fact we have arrived at Dive Site Number One: Aow Leuk, or Deep Bay. From here, we can see the rocky outcrop of Shark Island, where currents are strong, reef sharks linger and, I am told, massive whale sharks sometimes drift by.

I do my best to put those thoughts out of my head, and focus on what is happening where I am now. Being mindful. Being present. The kind of thing Mandi's Oxford CBT specialist might advise. I take a deep breath and peer past the fenders. The water is clear. I can see to the sand at the bottom. Shadows flit underneath us, distorted by the waves. As I pull on my fins, I watch Matt and Mina step off the back of the boat. They float in the water, giggling. And suddenly it's my turn.

I don't think I'm ready for this.

4

The Dive

'Decide whether you can make the dive safely. Remember: this is your decision . . .'

GENERAL OPEN WATER SKILLS,
PADI OPEN WATER MANUAL, 1999–2007

My first dive in the Gulf of Thailand is happening. Somehow it is happening right now. Terry is waiting for me. It's time to stand up and heave myself down to the back of the boat, carefully stepping one fin in front of the other, following his lead. The Korean team, Mina and Matt, have not long been swallowed up by the water, leaving only spurts and air bubbles behind them. As I stare out from the aft, this all seems sickeningly unavoidable.

If I step forward I have no idea what's going to come next. I don't know whether the dive will be good or bad. I don't know if there will be sharks. I can't spot fins, or fish, or teeth. Not yet. But if I stop I can go no further. I can't conquer my phobia, or become a person who enjoys things like swimming with dolphins. I can't be a true adventurer, or someone who Discovers New Worlds.

All I can see around me now is the ocean. It's beneath us and it's everywhere. It's deep and slick and restless. It won't give away any secrets. I want this space and hate this space. I know it feels nothing for me in return. I gaze out across the waves, and fizz with apprehension. Then Terry steps out and plummets in through the looking-glass sheen, feet first. I wait for him to rise up and swim out of the way. This he does quickly. Then he gives me the *OK* signal.

'In you get,' he says.

My molars are fusing together. Thanks to the constant horror reel that plays through my predictions, I know that any second now Terry will be yanked down under the surface by a bull shark. This shark will clamp its hulking jaws around his calf and tear away the muscle in one piece, leaving threads of skin that hang from his leg like shredded Cheesestrings. I know it will because I've seen the same thing happen to somebody else. I've watched their shredded Cheesestrings hang on YouTube.

Any second now, Terry will flail and struggle to reach the surface. He'll become the next Chrissie, *Jaws'* first victim. Happy, playful Chrissie who only wanted to skinny dip in the moonlight. Like Chrissie, he'll be tossed and pulled through the water on an inescapable trajectory, turned into a rubber doll that gasps and chokes and scream-gargles phrases like 'Help me!' and 'It hurts!' Later he will be found in a nest of crabs.

I wait. And so does Terry. Still bobbing. Now scratching his head.

'Your turn,' he says.

My turn.

Since no sharks have yet appeared, I step into position. Meanwhile Terry shouts instructions at me from the water. The reminders. *Regulator in. Heel of the hand on the mouthpiece,*

Georgie. Fingers on the mask. Yep. And the other hand on the weight belt. Hold it there. That's it. Is your BCD inflated? No? Yes? Just fill it up. Ready? OK. Come on. Big step. Nice, big step away from the boat.

What madness it is to step away from a boat in the sea. How many victims, how many drowned, would want to yell at me from the depths, 'No, woman! Stay on the deck!'

Yet I watch myself lift my right leg. My foot hovers over the water.

Big step away. Mind the back of the boat. You need to not hit the back of your head on the boat.

Big step.

Big jump.

Come on, Georgie. Jump.

I launch myself up.

Gravity pulls me right down.

Momentarily anchored to nothing my stomach levitates, stunned. Then my organs and I rush into the sea, heavy with metal, my eyes scrunched tight despite my mask's protection. The air in my BCD brings me back to the surface. I am in the water. Deep water. I am floating in the Gulf of Thailand. In the waters beside Death Island. Home to some 360 species of—

'Come on, then,' says Terry. 'Swim to me.'

Secure in the BCD, I turn on to my back and kick my way towards him. The water is warm. It slips around my neck. I see no fish yet. No shark fins.

As we float, Terry shows me how to wipe my mask so it is clearer. Copying him, I gather what little saliva I can and spit on to the inside lens, rub, rinse with the sea, grip tightly and don't let the mask go. At the same time, Terry reminds me of the things we're about to do. Underwater lessons and tricks. Boxes to tick. There seem to be so many. He reminds me of the signals. Reminds me not to do thumbs up when I actually mean *OK*. If I do, every time I do, I owe him a drink.

He reminds me to avoid the titan triggerfish. 'Those bastards can bite hard,' he says. 'If they go for you and I'm too far off stick your fin in its mouth and let it chew that. Then swim out of its territory.'

Oh God.

'OK?' says Terry. 'You look nervous.'

'No probs here,' I say.

'Sure?'

I force a fake grin. Give him two thumbs up.

'That's two beers on you then,' says Terry.

Oh God.

Chuckling, he points his thumb down. 'Let's descend.'

There's a lot of mirroring involved in dive signals. I need to show I understand by putting my thumb down too. It feels as if I am decreeing my own destruction. I let out the air from my BCD like we practised back at the hostel, and immediately I'm sinking, bubbling beneath this layer that separates what I know from what I don't. They call it controlled descent. They could call it drowning with air. The water covers my head and suddenly I'm diving. I'm in the blue. *I know what I'm doing*, I tell myself. *I've done this before. This is just like the pool but bigger. It's fine. It's fine. Keep breathing.*

The site of Aow Leuk is no more than 8 metres deep and the bottom is instantly visible. That's where we're headed. On the way down I equalise the pressure in my ears by shifting my jaw, same as I'd do on a train in a tunnel. This is no kind of tunnel, however. It's wide and expansive. It takes almost no time to reach the sandy floor, and I scuff the sand with my knees while I remember how to be buoyant. Suddenly, I notice there are fish around me. Not huge numbers of fish but more than I've seen since my panic attack in Australia.

There are rainbow-coloured fish with streaming tails; a species that's small and black with a white lacey print; inky urchins with spiny shells like underwater mines; chubby eye-less sea cucumbers. My insides retreat. I prepare for the worst – but nothing happens. Nothing is reacting to my intrusion. Somehow looking at them doesn't feel quite real. Nothing does, apart from the sound of my breathing, and the strange little pops and clicks inside my head. Terry signals to me to ask if I'm OK. *OK*, I reply with my fingers. I feel just about OK.

It's almost like I'm watching the sea on television, and not only because of the indifference of these fish. The mask has given me a screen. It directs my view. The water distorts the picture, and lures me into thinking this isn't quite reality. The breathing helps as well: the slow in-and-out. I concentrate on it, like the CBT folks might tell me to do if I'd actually stopped in my mania to consult them. I also focus on keeping close to Terry. There's no way I'm letting him leave me behind. Not that he's swimming fast. Or trying to lose me. Our pace is leisurely. Almost relaxed.

Light kicks propel me forward. As we make our way to an empty patch of sand, a golden-coloured butterfly fish approaches from the right, coming within inches of my face. I tense up but the fish could not care less. It doesn't look at me or open its mouth. I might as well be invisible: a rock, or another fish. The vibrant creature continues on its route to find food or a mate. Or perhaps it is just swimming to pass the time, enjoying the sensation of its movements. Later I read that these fish don't stray far from home – I might have been on its doorstep – and I'm even more impressed at its lack of fuss. For the moment, however, I carry on after Terry. My heartbeat is slowing. My panic feels muted. My own movements through the water feel *OK*.

Terry signals to check how much air I have left in my tank. I take a look at my gauge and give him the reply with my fingers. Every few minutes I check again, preparing myself for when he'll ask next. The practice keeps me busy. It gives me the illusion of control, something to focus on other than what might go wrong. From time to time, we go through one of our exercises. Pivots. Masks. Tows. I can't keep track of what they are or what I'm supposed to be doing, and I can't remember the signals. Instead I do what I think might be right and hope for an *OK*. Half the time I get it. Half the time I'm way off the mark, and shown something else to copy. I imagine this must be frustrating for Terry, but under the sea, peeping through his mask, his face takes on a far friendlier aspect than it's ever had towards me on the land. His eyes have grown gentle and wide. Plus there's no fag dangling out of his mouth. I wonder how the sea has transformed my own face. I wonder if I look friendly now, or fearful.

After what feels like no time at all, Terry turns to me and makes the signal for ascent: *thumbs up* and then *OK*. I copy him. *Thumbs up. OK.* Let's go. Multiple fish have passed me by now, including a large grey puffer with protruding marble eyes. This puffer passed me deflated, unthreatened, its spines flat on all sides.

Following Terry, recalling my training, I look up to the translucent roof of water 8 metres above us. Or perhaps I should think of it more as a roof of air. Whatever it is, we rise up slowly towards it, deflating our BCDs to counter the expansion of gases inside them as the pressure eases off. We each raise a hand, keeping watch for boats and their angry propellers. Better they slice up our wrists than our necks. Moments later, we break through and emerge into the light, inflating our BCDs, holding ourselves in the world of dry land and skies. When I check myself I appear to be alive. It would also appear that I've had no panic attacks. This feels like a promising start.

The boat picks us up and takes us to our second dive site of the day, a spot called Hin Ngam, further south, allowing us time to set up new tanks as we go. Again Matt and Mina dive first. Again I look out to Shark Island and wonder what waits for me there. But this time I walk to the water with a little less hesitation.

'Twelve metres down, this site,' preps Terry. 'More rocks and coral pinnacles.'

At Hin Ngam we stay under for forty-five minutes, and the world of the surface is conspicuously more distant. Creatures flit between the corals, and this time I struggle to work out my own dimensions, fearful of kicking chunks off anything living, or slicing myself on any one of the numerous jagged points in the vicinity. Clownfish – orange Nemos – peer out at me as I jerk past. I've heard that these little fish can sometimes bite divers, but from the safety of my television specs I bring myself to look at them regardless, observing sagging mouths and serious expressions. Not one of them tries to launch itself into my eyes. Or goes for my legs. My luck seems to be holding.

Among the set of exercises on this second training dive is one that forces me to cast off my regulator – the mouthpiece which enables me to breathe – throw it somewhere behind my shoulder, then set about calmly retrieving it. Suddenly I'm 12 metres deep in Thai waters with no air flowing freely into my lungs. It is the stuff of nightmares. If a shark comes now I'm done for. But I don't have time to let the panic soar. I do what I've been told and feel for the air hose. After some fumbling it leads me to what I need, and a hard puff clears the water from my reg. I can breathe again. Terry mimes applause, but all I can think is, *I'd never be that controlled if he wasn't here.*

At the end of the dive, Terry and I are the first to pull ourselves back on to the boat. Several minutes later Mina surfaces, as does Matt. She is bleeding, has cut her skin on some rock, and looks extremely unhappy. Having assisted her onto the boat, Matt announces to all onboard that Mina is the Barracuda Queen; that she spotted not only barracuda on their dive, but an unusual white moray eel. The two of them talk in a huddle as we make our way back to the harbour, instructor soothing student until she starts smiling again. I think of my clownfish. The marble-eyed puffer. I try to be pleased with what I've seen, but I can't make myself feel satisfied. Despite my phobic instincts, I start to wish I'd found a moray too – a slippery, glaring eel that lurches out of holes in rocks and wrecks. I also wish I'd seen a barracuda – the foil-shining fish with sharp fangs and a grim reputation. If I'd swum with a moray, I tell myself, if I'd shared the open water with barracuda, maybe I'd be able to shake off my fears more quickly. Maybe I'd be further along the road to coping with giant sharks.

I feel anxious to get down that road sharpish. Because tomorrow, for the final two dives I must pass before qualifying, we're heading to the 'star site' of Chumphon Pinnacle. According to my guidebook this is the best place in Koh Tao to encounter passing whale sharks, which means it is my best chance here to swim with the largest fish in all the world – to look my fear straight in the eye and see what looks back out. Only then can I move on, ready to live my new life.

Because of the prostitute incident with the Canadians, I've been transferred to my own room for my last night here on

Koh Tao, free of charge. More gratifying still, when I went to reception to officially lodge my complaint, I could see the main offender next to the pool – the man I referred to before as Canadian One. Like me, it seems, C-One is learning to scuba dive with PADI.

'THAT'S HIM,' I pointed, talking as loudly as I could. 'THAT'S THE MAN WHO TOOK A PROSTITUTE BACK TO OUR DORM ROOM LAST NIGHT.' C-One and I locked eyes. The sunbathers looked over their mobile phones.

The receptionist said, 'Oh.'

When I get back to the hostel from diving Hin Ngam, I settle into my sheets and finally feel a gladdening sense of achievement. Not only have I made it through my first dives and fish encounters without dying, successfully completing the initial steps of my phobia elimination programme, but now, instead of having to sleep in a stuffy, cramped dorm, I get a twin room with fans, TV, patio area, en suite and bar of soap to myself. It's all to be added to the Canadian's own bill. This time tomorrow I'll be shot of him, Death Island, Terry and his cigarettes. I'll have ridden a boat to Koh Pha-Ngan, and will be resting on a beach with cocktails. Working through the checklist. Tick, tick, tick.

When I wake up the following day it takes me only seconds to realise that things have gone badly wrong. My journal for Granny records the morning as follows:

What was supposed to happen this a.m.:
6.40 – wake up
7.20 – leave for Chumphon Pinnacle
10.45 (approx.) – swim with whale shark and conquer phobia for ever
12.00 – return from Chumphon Pinnacle

14.00 – bus to ferry
15.00 – ferry to Pha-Ngan
16.10 – arrive Pha-Ngan
16.30 – check in to pre-booked hotel on the beach.
Relaxation stations.

What actually happened this morning:
7.33 – wake up
7.34 – throw on clothes and run
7.35 – find Terry on a chair with our unloaded
kit. Truck left 15 minutes ago. Miss boat for
Chumphon Pinnacle.

I am furious with myself. Boiling with despair. It's the first time I've ever slept through an alarm, and all thanks to the comfort of a bed I shouldn't have been in. Now I'll have to miss the ferry I've already paid for. The hotel I've already paid for. I'll have to fork out more money and stay on Koh Tao for an extra night, or I can't even complete the last part of my training.

I work hard for a while to unclench my fists, but making them stay that way is harder. Then worse news makes itself known to me. Because I've missed the morning boat, Terry explains, sucking on an early cigarette, I'll have to take my final Open Water dives this afternoon. This afternoon the boat won't be making its way back to Chumphon Pinnacle. Instead it'll be going somewhere else, somewhere with a much smaller chance of whale sharks. And travelling in the boat with us: who else but my friend, Canadian Number One.

I ask Terry if there's any way of doing my last dives tomorrow instead, on a boat without the Canadian.

'Nope,' he says, barely hiding his smile. 'I'm not instructing tomorrow. If you don't want to dive this afternoon you can wait until I get back in a few days' time, or leave on your ferry this afternoon without qualifying.'

Leave in the afternoon without qualifying . . . The thought is tempting. If I head to Pha-Ngan this afternoon I won't have to see the Canadian ever again. And I won't have to stay on this island surrounded by back-packing teens and secret murderers. Then I think, *If I do leave now, what exactly have I accomplished on this trip to Koh Tao?* Discovering I can swim in the water with clownfish and not black out is not quite the triumph I wanted.

There are also financial elements to consider. This Open Water qualification alone has cost me in excess of £400. That's not counting the transport I took to get here. The flights to Bangkok. The flights from Bangkok. The ferry from the mainland. My job.

And as my gaze darts from palm fronds, to deserted pool, to empty dive school forecourt, it starts to really sink in that I left my job to come here. Because I wanted to conquer my fear. Because my life of concrete and daily routines lacked excitement. Because I wanted to gather new stories. Because I wanted a purpose that didn't involve acquiring a mortgage. Because I thought I wanted more than a fucking job.

My permanent, highly respectable, fucking job.

My only fucking source of fucking income.

My heart sinks. It can't have all been for clownfish. I need pride. I need adventure. I need a harpoon-free version of *Moby-Dick*. I need to slay the fear that is my monster. I want awe, damn it. A tale that'll blow Granny's mind.

I want a whole new attitude to life.

Fighting to sound calm, to keep my voice steady, I tell Terry I'll be there to dive with him after lunch. And off I go back to my bastard, fan-cooled bedroom.

After pacing the floor for some time, I stop to scribble notes in a rage, picturing Mina and Matt on their way to the dive site. The site that's widely agreed to be one of the best in the Gulf of Thailand. They're on their way there. At this very moment. I picture the two of them sinking into the water and meeting a fully grown whale shark within a few seconds of their submergence. I watch Mina's sense of wonder grow behind her mask, expanding to match the size of the fearsome creature that swims beside her. I can see the almost religious experience of it; disbelief overridden by evidence: there *can't* be a fish that big, a mouth that wide and that dark, and yet here it all is, swimming by, straight out of a fairy tale and beside her slender frame, opening up like a black hole at the edge of a distant galaxy. To have proof that this mythical fantasy creature *exists*.

I imagine the intensity of the moment. Of witnessing that that there is something far, far greater than yourself. Greater than your daily routine. Greater than any job. The sensation of confronting your own insignificance, and of finding it overwhelming. Of being held in place by the currents, then swept to one side by a tail the size of a steeple. Of emerging back into the air above, a survivor.

I think so hard about all these things that I give myself physical pain. I feel like if I stay in my room and continue to think like this, I'm going to turn blue.

Disappointment and I do not mix well.

I have to get out. I take a deep breath, yell into my pillow, cover my face with sun cream and leave the room. The whale shark won't show this morning, I tell myself, part-walking, part-stamping my feet, towards the shore. And when the whale shark comes this afternoon I'll hide behind Terry and watch it eat the Canadian. That's right. Phobia or no phobia, I wouldn't want to miss that for the world.

Though it's barely nine in the morning the humidity is

already unbearable. I stay by the coastline, craning my neck for a breeze and finding nothing. I don't know where I'm heading, but I keep going. My back aches from carrying thick aluminium cylinders. My hips ache from the kilos of lead I've been stringing along my belt. My throat and lips are dry from sucking in bottles of compressed air. But still I want to go far. I want to walk until I forget all of my problems; forget that I missed Koh Tao's best dive site by fifteen unconscious minutes. Perhaps I can sweat out my residual anger. If stress is a flight-or-fight response, I'm flying as far as my water bottle takes me.

That point turns out to be the end of the road, in a very literal sense. I pass through a hollow of trees to a beach resort and at once I can go no further. There's a small sign for a snorkelling spot, so I follow it down a flight of wooden steps and emerge across the bay from the two humps of Nang Yuan island. On the other side of those humps, north-west within the Gulf, is Chumphon Pinnacle.

I need to stop myself thinking before I want to yell again, so I strip off my shirt and shorts, and stand by the water's edge in my swimsuit. Close by is a school of small, bright yellow fish, plus a few pieces of coral and other flora. It's an opportunity for a training session. Let's see how far I've progressed.

'I can do small, bright yellow fish now,' I say to myself. 'I can do coral and flora.' Adjusting the strap of my goggles across my hair – I have no mask or snorkel – I step into the sea. The school of fish gathers around my legs. I let them hover. *Breathe in. Breathe out. These fish are nothing but harmless leaves in the wind.* I pull my goggles over my nose and prepare to float above them. Before my feet have time to leave the ground I have been bitten.

The shock of it sends me shooting straight back to my heap of rumpled clothes. There I stand and pant. *Oh God oh God oh God.* I've been poisoned. My first trip to Thailand and I've been killed by a fish that's cartoonishly yellow and small. I examine my shin where I felt the bite. I prod and stretch the skin. There's no mark there at all. No blood. When I calm down I notice it doesn't even hurt.

I tell myself this is all part of the training. Surely that's what the Oxford CBT lot would say. Which means there's nothing else to do but re-enter the water. Time to get back on the seahorse.

'Fuck you, bright yellow fish.' It's hot. I'm sweaty. I've had a bad morning. Right now I need to swim and not freak out.

This time I don't bother planting my feet on the sand. Instead I splash over the school as fast as I can. To my surprise the fish don't follow, and I'm able to paddle towards a shallow reef where I feel more untouchable. Here I'm a casual observer again, some kind of peeping Tom. It's my goggles, I think. Like the diving mask, they give me the sense of being at one remove from the action. I notice a cluster of needlefish: silver creatures with narrow bodies and long, pointed jaws. They're metallic, scaled-down animals, alligator-esque. A lump of nerves heaves from my chest to my throat. But when they see my approach the needlefish dart away and don't come back. Aha. I am powerful now. Almost safe.

As soon as a bulky yellow and purple fish darts into the path of my eyeline, however, that sensation of safety gushes out of me. Four prominent front teeth protrude from its lips. The thing looks mean, and I recognise it. This is a titan triggerfish. The species that aggressively attacks anything which enters the zone above its eggs. The one with the nasty bite. It's suddenly clear why the bright yellow school didn't follow me this way.

I think that's enough solo training for now.

*

A few hours later I'm suited up and ready for my last two Koh Tao dives. The Canadian sits on the opposite side of the boat. He is glaring at me, saying nothing. Never mind that oversleeping was technically my fault. This arsehole caused the chain of events that kept me from Chumphon Pinnacle this morning. If it wasn't for him and his sexual urges I'd be on my way to the pier and an evening of caipirinhas on Pha-Ngan. If it wasn't for him I'd be Open Water qualified already. I would have coped with a whale shark by now.

I glare right back.

Under the surface we stay well away from each other. It's just Terry and me, ticking the last of the boxes at 18 metres, the maximum depth I can do with this level of training: maintaining neutral buoyancy so I can hover; removing my mask, replacing it and clearing the water out with a snort of my nose; pulling the tip of my fins towards me as I would need to do if I had cramp in my legs. In between tasks I follow Terry, check my air and scan the water for predators and whale sharks. There is only a large school of young barracuda, forming an ominous cloud in the distance. They stay in formation and keep away.

On my second and final training dive I see my first moray, a crotchety-looking eel which opens and closes its jaws as if silently whining. On my own I would be paralysed. But Terry points towards it, then passes by, unaffected. The moray seems to follow his progress with interest, poking its head from the coral and watching with white zombie eyes. But it doesn't come out of its hole. And it's smaller than I expected. I move a little further out and the moray lets me pass after Terry without taking issue.

As the dive boat carries us back to the mainland, I toy with the idea that I've cured myself of my phobia already. Perhaps I don't need the giant shark after all. Four dives with fish, plus an incident of biting, and no loss of my faculties has occurred. To prove my theory I put my brain to work. I think of the steady sway of a reef shark. The intelligent eye of a dolphin. A suspended wall of jellyfish, their tentacles like plastinated nerves. I see the mammoth shadow of the whale shark, emerging slowly out from the limitless blue.

The blood in my face, chest and thighs flushes cold.

'Why are whale sharks your goal?' a diver asks me later. 'If this is about fear of fish, why not aim to conquer your fear by swimming with one of the scarier ones that could actually do some damage?'

I mull this question over for a while, unable to think of an answer. Afterwards, too late, I think about what I could have said: that I'm not stupid enough to jump in with great whites; that this is a form of therapy, after all, not a suicide mission. But it's not the only reason whale sharks suit my plan, I realise. It is what the whale shark represents – what every fear, at its core, is all about.

Imagine the scene as I often do.

Imagine you find yourself in a vast body of deep water with no visible edges. Not a single one. This body of water stretches further than you can ever comprehend.

Imagine being suspended in this water, nothing to see above the waves apart from the sky and the sides of your nose.

Imagine that you have been split in two, from the neck down. On the surface you are a fleshy, useless head and noth-ing else. Salty water prickles your skin. You are a body part barely floating, and that's all. Beneath the line of water which cuts across your throat, everything else is hidden. You cannot be sure of what's there. Your feet are in another place. As are your thighs. Your torso. Your heart.

In some ways it would be easier if you lay on the water's

surface and floated, but that would mean turning your back on what's underneath you. Because although this water seems clear when it's cupped in your hands, you cannot see much through the layer that cloaks your neck. And you know, you just know, that something is on its way up to you.

It is watching.

Approaching.

And you know that you need to be ready when it comes.

Imagine that the dark blue water around you slowly turns black. Imagine that this thing has now arrived. And imagine, for the first time you have ever known, that you are tiny. The tiniest thing you can see. So small that you could be sucked into this creature's open mouth and swallowed whole.

The whale shark isn't just a fish. The whale shark is death itself.

5

Dark Places

'Diving should be personal.'

CONTINUING YOUR ADVENTURE,
PADI OPEN WATER MANUAL, 1999–2007

I know the end is coming. It's waiting in the water. Doesn't matter how skilled you are at swimming, or how many PADI certifications you acquire. One day, perhaps when you're most confident it won't, death will appear. This is the message I hear if I stop ignoring what I'm trying to ignore.

Things like the rest of the conversation I had with Alex, the swim-averse diving instructor back in England – the parts of it that weren't telling me I could conquer my fears with diving and go far. In that conversation, Alex also told me that a competent student of his had drowned in the water last summer. He couldn't share all the details, he said. The inquest was still ongoing. What he could say is that it was a freak accident. And that being there while it happened was horrible.

Before it happened, losing a student was one of Alex's worst nightmares. 'I think that's always been something that's been a fear,' he said to me, 'because you feel that if you get into the water enough times, eventually you're going to be unlucky enough to be there when it goes wrong.'

Another diver I chatted with also spoke candidly about the shock of seeing her friend's drowned body at his funeral. She told me that his head was swollen, distorted by the water. She told me that this is what happens to victims of drowning.

The image sticks. I never knew drowning victims had swollen heads. That water could seep so quickly in through the membranes of our bodies, filling our veins until they burst. Lifting our skin and flooding the gaps beneath. Making our eyes wide and bulbous. Turning us into strange fish.

Until these conversations, I'd always thought of drowning as old-fashioned, an experience exclusive to the past. There were times, long ago, when Granny Codd and I would sit on the promenade by the beach, looking out at the horizon, eating orange Soleros in the shade. While swatting at wasps we would watch people splash in the shallows, and compete to point out all the worst cases of sunburn. But if we ever saw anyone swimming towards the buoy, this game would suddenly stop. Then Granny Codd would tell me about the mornings she'd watched men drown near Bournemouth Pier. They would always be young, and swimming to boast to their friends. As she watched they'd succumb to cramp far away from the shore, and slip under the surface where they died before help could reach them.

Granny Codd has spent most of her life by the sea, growing up in and out of boats and beach huts. But she can't stand being in the water. She has seen too many swollen heads, and not just at the pier. One beautiful day when she was a child, she walked to Poole's large harbour, wanting to cross to the beach on the other side. Searching for a way over, she spotted a boat that looked right for the job. It had very recently returned to shore. Its oars were wet and glistening. Granny was excited. She stepped into it just as the harbourmaster shouted at her to steer clear. Inside she found a man who had apparently fallen asleep along the hull. His skin was purple.

Decades later, during a short writing class, she wrote part of the episode into a poem. I remember finding that poem on the bookshelf; the moment its young narrator says to the harbourmaster, 'Shh, you will wake that man.'

'Him?' the harbourmaster responds.

He won't wake; he's dead. Drowned. That's what you'll be if you don't look where you're going.

And the moral is: Be focused. Beware. Never underestimate the sea.

When I was no longer a child, but still some years ago – before she entered the nursing home and her mind started to falter – Granny shared another story with me. She told me that, during the Second World War, she received an unexpected telegram from the army. It informed her that her husband, the one true love of her life, had drowned off the coast near Beirut. Not long after that, Granny slashed her wrist in her sleep. She unconsciously grabbed a blade within reach – one she used for dress alterations – and woke to find she was bleeding into the sheets. When asked, she would roll up her shirt sleeves and show me the scars. Somewhere there's a poem about that too. One day I hope to find it.

In the meantime I can't help thinking: had her first husband come back alive from Lebanon, my grandmother would not have married again, and ended up with the man who'd become my grandfather. She would not have been Granny Codd. None of the Codds in my family would have been born. Because a sergeant drowned in the sea, I exist. He was my age when he died. Like me, he had grown up swimming. I wonder if he ever felt afraid as he waded in.

The World Health Organization (WHO) describes drowning as the 'third leading cause of unintentional death worldwide,' behind only road traffic accidents and falls. In 2015, the WHO has estimated, 360,000 people died from drowning. In certain areas of the world – what the WHO calls the Western Pacific Region – drowning is the leading cause of death for children aged five to fourteen. And of all the people who drown every year on our planet, the one- to four-year-old age group makes up the highest proportion of the statistics.

When I mentioned I was planning to learn to dive, that I was fearful of what might happen down there, my uncle Jon, Granny Codd's second-born, told me a story I'd not heard before. He described how, when he was a toddler, his older sister convinced him to climb the side of a large water butt in their back garden. It had been left there by builders who were fixing up the house. As soon as he reached the top my uncle tumbled in. He couldn't swim. Luckily his sister, my eldest aunt Josie, called out to fetch the adults. He was rescued.

Jon told me that this incident happened so early in his life he couldn't remember it. Moreover, he'd grown up unafraid of swimming – in fact, he and his wife were the only scuba divers in my family. Then Jon went on to tell me about how he feels when he enters the water to dive: how the instant his face meets the surface his breaths grow frantic and shallow. How it takes him a moment to calm himself down before he can continue.

His wife, who was talking with us, spoke up to say she had the same reaction. Together they made joint noises of agreement, talking about their responses as if they were commonplace. I waited for it to happen to me on my first dives. It didn't.

But perhaps it should be happening. Perhaps that would be useful. What would be more rational: to be put off diving

early, like the people who know just how bad the water can
be, or to carry on swimming towards the big fish – continuing deeper into a realm of disaster?

Koh Tao, David the art dealers' son, the Canadians – a ferry
ride puts all of them behind me. Terry too, a man I disliked,
but ultimately trusted with my life. I am left now with only
a signed diver's log book to prove our time together.

From where I am currently based, on the neighbouring island
of Koh Pha-Ngan, I should be able to dive again – I still have
time to do it before Ted gets here. But instead of banishing
fears like I want to, I've spent the past four nights contending
with the worst stomach bug I've ever known. Someone has
replumbed my bowel as a rusty water fountain. Every time I feel
it creaking on, I hobble to sit on the toilet and wince. I think
back to the 'fresh' Thai desserts I bought from the local night
market on my first evening here; flavours I'd planned to report
back on for Granny. Sweet. Lukewarm. Sulphurous.

I had thought about visiting Sail Rock from Pha-Ngan and
travelling to the Gulf's top dive site – a 'veritable beacon for
whale sharks', according to my guidebook. But when I muster
the strength to risk leaving the bathroom I sit in an internet
café instead, scrawling on postcards, then logging in for Ted's
updates on London life – the people coming to look for a disappeared neighbour; rumours of a brothel in the second floor
of our block; the lurid new trainers he's ordered to go in his
suitcase – all the while replenishing my stomach with salty
crisps and fresh coconuts. Locals I've asked about Sail Rock say
the whale sharks haven't passed through in a while. A couple
of weeks ago one group saw a juvenile, just a few metres long.
But there's been nothing else since then. More surprisingly
still, even Mina and Matt had no luck at Chumphon Pinnacle.

I am told the Andaman Sea should bring better fortunes.

Out there is a place called Richelieu Rock, where whale sharks can be spotted at this time of year. Perhaps by the time I get there my body will have stopped rebelling against me. And perhaps, by then, more therapy will have eased my fears of big fish. For now the only prep I can do is cross my fingers and hold off on the Thai sweets.

It's a painful journey back to the mainland by boat, then across the south peninsula to Khao Lak. I clamber down from the bus in the late afternoon, more than seven hours after I started the journey, and emerge on to a busy road which ultimately wends south to Phuket. This is the heart of Khao Lak: a noisy, unattractive strip of dive shops, bars, cheap cafés, hotchpotch restaurants and souvenir stores. It's not until after I leave that I realise the town had previously been flattened, and at least 3950 people killed, by the Boxing Day tsunami that struck here in 2004. Though you wouldn't know it from this section of road, Khao Lak is the leaping-off spot for the Andaman. Right now it's hard to tell the sea is even near – those views are reserved for resort guests only. Oblivious to the ghosts around me, I make my job finding a place to stay, and working out how to get to Richelieu.

On a cheap bed in a newly opened hostel, I plot my next steps. If I am to make myself properly ready for whale sharks, I will probably need to spend a few days on the ocean before we meet. And that would make this the best place to be. Khao Lak is the home of the Andaman liveaboard: multiple operators taking multiple divers out to 'live aboard' a boat for multiple days and multiple dives. Many nights at sea means many chances to acclimatise – and many chances to swim with the world's biggest fish.

Physically, I'm feeling a little more stable than I was on Pha-Ngan, so I lock up my backpack and head out to eat. I

will need to properly fill my stomach before I can contemplate liveaboards. But I haven't been away from the hostel
for even five minutes when I'm drawn to a shop showing
footage of a diver swimming with what looks to me like a
fully grown, behemoth whale shark.

Despite the small screen the shark seems huge; the diver
an insect beside it. Seeing the two of them float in the blue
makes my skin bristle and shrink – imagine being that close
to totally losing your sense of self – though content-wise it's
nothing like the whale shark attack video I've watched on
YouTube time and time again. The shark here isn't antsy. It's
just hovering. Sucking gulps near the surface while the diver
looks on. I wonder who this diver is. What they're thinking.
What the whale shark is thinking. What happens after this
video stops and loops back to the beginning?

Mega sea beasts circle in my mind. Thanks to my empty
stomach, and having rattled across the country in a bus, I lack
the strength and know-how to contain them. I cannot get
rid of my fears if I can't find a way to confront them. I stick
my head inside the shop and hear myself say to the woman
inside, 'I need to get to Richelieu Rock. Are you running
any liveaboard trips tomorrow?' Then I hear myself asking:
'How much?'

Plunging into this new mission, I pose the same two questions to every dive shop proprietor along the strip and quickly
get into a bargaining situation. A fat dive shop rep holds a
clutch of liveaboard leaflets, wipes the sweat from his forehead and drops another 1000 baht from his very-best-final
offer. The room is full of people. On every flat surface stand
reps in identical T-shirts, either passing pens and contracts to
divers, or counting up the cash. The next ship leaves tonight,
in three hours' time to be precise, and there's only one space
left. That space could be mine, he says. The trip would entail

fourteen dives in total. In two days they'll be doing a day of four dives at Richelieu alone. And on the way they'll stop at a place called Koh Bon, where the giant mantas live.

'More than 6 metres,' he says, throwing his arms open. 'Big, *big* fish.'

The leaflets tremble under a ceiling fan, agitated by the breeze. I see myself pull out the credit card from my pocket. I seem to be buying a place on the boat, my last few hundred pounds of spending money thrown in to the cause. Actual therapy with an actual therapist would have been dramatically cheaper. Better put that thought back in its box: I'm already too far gone. My right leg judders, separate from the rest of me. The dive rep sweats and lays out all the paperwork, tapping the large sum into his card machine as I skim through pages of terms and conditions. *Damage, loss, injury, death.* I pass the card over and he pushes it into the slot. Now I'm typing in the pin. Am I? This all feels rather sudden.

The card machine blurps. It sounds angry. Declined.

'Have you got another card?' he asks. 'Cash?'

'Try it again,' I say. Perhaps my finger slipped. I must have entered the wrong pin.

We try it again. Declined. Now my left leg is juddering too.

'Hold that place for me,' I say. 'I'll go get cash. Five minutes. Where's the ATM?'

I run out to the street and launch myself on to the main road, lunging through gaps in the traffic until I find it. Shaking with adrenaline I insert my card and wait for a response; punch in the pin. I get to the balance but it won't let me take out my money. I pound the floor with my sandal.

I need to call the bank, but don't have a phone. I need to find a phone. There must be a phone here somewhere. Except I might not be able to pay for it. If I pay for the phone I won't have enough cash left to buy my food. Then again, if the phone call works, I'll be on a boat eating dinner in a few hours' time. If it doesn't work there'll be no food *and* no money.

I argue with myself for minutes, eventually deciding I can go without food. But after hurrying up and down the shops in a fruitless search for a public telephone that, as usual, doesn't exist, I realise this isn't going to work. And maybe it shouldn't. Maybe I should calm down and buy some dinner, like I intended to do when I left my hostel room an hour ago. *Less throwing yourself into roads, Georgie. More eating of food.*

The next day it takes a full morning of touring hotel lobbies, pleading with receptionists, emailing Ted from my hostel's computer, and following rumours of borrowable mobile phones, to find the means of contacting my bank and sorting my cash-flow crisis. In the heat of midday, exhausted with all humanity – the chief representative of the species being me at this moment in time – I hire a bike with my new-found cash and cycle to a nearby national park; an effort to switch off my brain and lower the tension. At the park I find bizarre marine creatures clumsily flipping themselves from the sea and all over the rocks. They look like a mixture of leech and sea slug, with suckers at either end of their pencil-length bodies. I have never seen anything like them, nor have any of the people who pass by. I can only think they are aliens trying to colonise Planet Earth, and I watch from a distance until it gets too creepy. Then I hurry off to the nearest beach. I never do discover what they are.

After draining the contents of a coconut well away from any rocks, I return to the town for a less hectic tour of the dive shops. In spite of my aim to stay cool and think things through, I'm instantly drawn into another feverish bargaining process. Any power I had yesterday over my guy with the sweat and leaflets has evaporated. Now that I've come back to him, he knows I need his services more than he needs me. His rates have become sticky. I scurry off elsewhere, leaving the factory of signing divers behind me, and slip into a new shop recommended by my guidebook. It's quiet in here, and a French woman asks if she can help. Her voice conveys an inner calm I've never had myself. In the course of our conversation I learn that her company has limited spaces remaining on a liveaboard leaving this evening. It's been specially chartered by a group of Spanish I.T. specialists, and will not only include a whole day of diving at Richelieu and two dives at Koh Bon, but also a special set of dives at the Surin Islands – a rarity on liveaboards from these parts. That's five days instead of the usual four. There will even be an instructor onboard who can coach me as a new PADI diver. And because it's such late notice, because I'd be taking up space that would otherwise go untaken, they'll let me join for less than two-thirds of the price the others have paid.

'What about whale sharks?' I ask her.

'It's the right time of year,' she replies.

This is clearly a sales pitch designed to reel in impulsive fools like me. But I also feel that right now I have no better option. It's either stay in Khao Lak with marauding leech-slugs, numbing my disappointment with pancakes and cocktails until Ted's flight is due, or blow the last of my diving budget and finally go where the whale sharks are. I reach into my pocket for my card.

Hours later, I'm standing on the bridge of the liveaboard watching fire spew out all over the prow, plugging my ears against a series of explosions. The firecrackers have been lit, and are marking our blazing departure. As we pull away from the dock, one of the crew sees a cat that has crept onboard. Without hesitation he picks it up and lobs it over the widening gulf as if it's another firework. The cat reaches the jetty without blowing up, and toddles away in a daze.

Alone again, back in my cabin, the combination of nerves
and engine noises keeps me wide awake. We are motoring overnight to the Similan Islands. Heading straight for whale sharks.
In desperation I take one of the pills that were recommended
to me by my now-ex boss, a urological surgeon. Hearing me
complain about being incapable of sleep while on the move, and
learning about the weeks of long-haul travelling I was giving
up his employ to undergo, he wrote me out a prescription for
something that would 'really do the job. Journeys without this
stuff? Just horrific. Don't waste your time with Diazepam.' I
lie back on my pillow, waiting for the tiredness to take over,
like it did when I popped the first on my outward flight. After
a few minutes my stomach tingles. *Yes*, I think. *Come on, sleep.*

Ted.

The job.

Granny.

Drowning.

Death.

The fish.

The sea.

The shark.

Half an hour later, I'm still wide awake. If Ted were around
he'd rub my nose until I fell asleep. If only he would appear.
Missing him keenly, I pop another pill. Then one more just to
be sure. In exhausted distress I smother my face with a pillow.
Eventually the cabin around me turns black.

I come to a little while later. The engines are off and the sun
is up. My watch says it's almost time for breakfast. Upstairs,
over slivers of fake white bread and quivering hillocks of jam,
I sit with some of the other early risers, and hear that a few of
these divers haven't been underwater for years – unless you
count their recent refreshers in the pool. Some of them are
nervous. They're also not all Spanish I.T. specialists: one of the

party is a Danish woman, Liv (pronounced *l-yuh*), who was smuggled aboard last-minute just like me. Liv is a veritable babe, with an Elvis tattoo on her upper thigh, and wearing the length of short shorts needed to keep all but the top of the King's quiff on full display. Over the last few weeks she's gone from unqualified diver to fully advanced with PADI, and she can't stop grinning at the prospect of what lies ahead. It would appear that Thailand's been transformative for her in more ways than one. When she arrived in the country her hair was its natural dark brown, almost black. Right now it's bright blonde. All thanks to the sun, she says – and she seems like such a charmed woman that I can believe her.

It's not long before we're receiving our first briefing of the trip, and I'm linked with Andrew, a British diving instructor with a side-swept, boy-band-style fringe. Andrew doesn't smell of smoke, and knows how to smile without cynicism. Things are looking up for me already. Accompanied by a detailed whiteboard diagram, he stands and explains to all the divers assembled what we need to know – where we are, which route we'll take on the dive, how deep we can go, who's with which instructor, what creatures to look out for – no word of a whale shark or manta just yet. By 8.02 a.m., he and I are in the water, descending. There's no time to panic or question what I'm doing. I'm just doing it. In crystal clear water. Over a reef.

Also on this reef, I soon discover, is a giant moray eel. Keeping close to Andrew, I watch its head – a head that's not far off the size of my own – snake out from a gap in the reef wall. The stalk of its saggy, corpse-like neck hovers opposite us in the current, before the rest unspools into open water. The serpentine length of its body coils and bends. It must be at least a couple of metres long. Maybe longer. But, praise be, it's heading in the opposite direction. I keep breathing.

I must keep breathing.

Later a lionfish crosses our path and we steer clear of its billowing, venomous spines, with their power to cause great pain, breathing problems and convulsions – not to mention, in some cases, temporary paralysis and heart failure. Like the eel, the lionfish makes it clear that it has no interest in us, and I'm able to watch it flutter through the water without freaking myself out. To admire its beauty, even. It's almost as if the immersion has sedated me.

Two more gentle dives take us into the late afternoon, and with no hint of whale sharks around I can feel myself unwinding. I can barely believe that it's happening, but a resistance to my phobia seems to be growing. It must be. How else could I share the water with a giant moray and a lionfish, and come back to the surface in one piece? Perhaps the smaller things and I are fine now. The bigger ones though – the ones large enough to cancel me out with their shadows – the thought of things like that still makes me tense. I know that in not too long a while I will be pitting myself against them. But not yet. Whale shark time is Richelieu Rock, I've decided. No need to think about monsters until then.

On the liveaboard, Andrew is setting up for the next briefing, drawing an intricate, marker-pen sketch of a new underwater world. I take a seat and flick through a guide to Andaman fish species. The whale shark, *Rhincodon typus*, looms out of the page like a zeppelin.

'How many of these have you dived with so far?' I ask. I hold the picture out to Andrew, turning it fully away from my face. Already I know that my newest instructor has taught diving in Thailand long enough to have found his own home here, as well as a committed local girlfriend. Which is why it surprises me all the more to see him grimace now.

'There was one trip we ran not long ago,' he says. 'A whale shark turned up then ...'

'Yes?'

'It was on my day off.'

I look at him. 'You've been diving here for years, right?'

'Yep.'

'And you've never seen a whale shark.'

'Nope.'

'Shit.'

'Yep. It is.'

From that moment on, I notice how much Andrew devotes himself to extolling the virtues of micro diving to me – that is, looking out for the smallest things on the reef, instead of the biggest. Nudibranchs, for example (sounds like 'nudie branks', not 'nudie branches'), which are a variety of dinky molluscs coming in thousands of crazy shapes and insanely bright colours. Looking through pictures of nudibranchs is like looking at a window display of chic, bijou erotica. I'm trying to imagine it, but I don't think sharing the water with these multicoloured sex toys is going to help me master my more major phobic responses.

Diving at night, on the other hand, might be a useful addition to my armoury. Not seeing, after all, feeds into so much fear. The scary movies that don't show the ghouls are always the most terrifying. The shapes beneath the water. The purple man just out of view.

Everyone knows that the sea is a riskier entity during the night. The surface, once transparent beneath the sun, offers even fewer clues to its contents when dark skies take over. What's left is an inky black. And a radically altered environment. The dark does things to sea creatures. Diurnal inhabitants enter a state that seems to resemble sleep. Certain species – the Spanish hogfish, for example; a bright, grazing wrasse that lives in the Western Atlantic – become totally motionless. They can even, I've heard, be pulled up to the surface without being woken. Large-eyed creatures, on the other hand, spring to life. Jumbo squid rise from the depths. Several species of shark lose their daytime sluggishness. Horn sharks, swell sharks, nurse sharks, tiger sharks. They embark on a new hunt.

'We'd usually only open night dives up to Advanced PADI divers,' Andrew tells me, 'but if you want to join in you can. Just don't drop your torch.' And so it is that, as the sun sinks over the dreamy white sand bay beside our mooring – a bay that Liv's instructor, Kwan, assures us is made of digested coral (a.k.a. 'fish shit') – the eighth dive of my life is set to take place in the moonlight.

There's a hammering in my chest as we divers congregate on the lowest level of deck. Here, at the back, the crew direct us to our kit and refilled tanks. They help us into our wet-suits, and secretly tie our long zips together, twinning us at the neck – something Liv and I don't notice until we move off for our checks. We are pinned at the throat until they release us. (James Deane and Paul would approve.)

Next everyone is given a torch, and told to secure it safely to their wrists. On a night dive no other diver can see your hands unless you light them up, so the usual gestures morph into something new:

- *OK* involves tracing a circle of light.
- *Attention* involves moving the torch straight up and down, or quickly shaking the beam.
- *Emergency* involves shining the light side-to-side.
- Pointing the light directly at someone else's face involves blinding them. Don't do it.

I step cautiously into the water and float between the station-ary boat's propellers, feeling my mind strain to separate from my body. I would love it if my emotions would just retreat – the angst especially – but, as usual, they cling on. I try focusing on the detail of every action I must do; ease myself apart from my mind in that way. I know that, if I don't, I'll start thinking about the unthinkable. At least Andrew is with me, as is Liv.

Torches on, we let our lights hang towards the seabed. First, we will attempt to stimulate phosphorescence. The black water closes above our heads and we half-sink, half-swim to the sea floor, 12 metres beneath where we're berthed. *This is not happening*, I decide. *My body is not me.* At the bottom, Andrew gives the signal for torches off. As briefed, we begin to swish our hands in the water. The eyes that aren't quite mine squint hard to see something, anything, when a small flash of blue glints back at them. It's like the light of a police car, far away. Black. Blue twinkle. Black.

When the torches come back on, a semi-transparent pattern is clustering around my hands and face. It is not a trick of the light, but a small group of tiny planktonian shapes. They have my full attention. Mystified, I move from side to side, lift my arm, flick my fingers at them. They follow my movements. I laugh. At this depth, filtered through a respirator, the laugh comes back to my ears like the sound of an old woman choking in the bath. When my mind really gets going, when I wonder what these plankton are really doing and why they're doing it, I start to wonder if they're even plankton at all. I always thought plankton were the oceanic equivalent of pollen. Or dust. Or mould. Not creatures that could firstly sense, and then track, a human hand. Are these the marine equivalent of dandelion seeds? Or are they sinister micro-stalkers?

Maybe they're sea mosquitoes. I once read about sea mosquitoes in a Cousteau book about sharks. Two of Cousteau's crew, Goupil and Tomasi, were night-diving in a shark cage between Yemen and Djibouti when they dropped their cameras, behaving as if possessed. Jacques Cousteau, who watched the scene from afar, wrote that, 'little white dots were swirling around them ... The human silhouettes inside the cage were twisting into every imaginable shape, as if seized by a sudden madness.' They aborted the dive and took their cage to the surface. Cousteau followed them up.

The scene when he arrived on the after deck was a troubling one: it was deserted, Cousteau wrote, and 'covered with blood stains'. He hurried to the officers' mess to discover Goupil and Tomasi lying on tables, being tended to by the ship's doctor, and wracked with pain. 'There were spots of blood on the floor, on the tables, and even on the partitions,' he wrote. His friends had been the victims of minute, near-invisible flesh-eating crustaceans: sea mosquitoes, maybe thousands of them. Each had lost more than a pint of blood. They had both been protected by wetsuits, except for the narrow gaps between their suit legs and their fins. It was all the mosquitoes needed.

A pint of blood each. From their ankles. I jerk away from the white shapes before me, feeling my skin prickle, and realise I'm quite a distance from the others. Now, as well as jolting my limbs at hypothetical wraiths and parasites, I need to catch up with a spectral duo of lights. Haven't Liv and Andrew noticed I'm missing? Maybe that's why they're speeding up. *See how well that nervy one copes when she's alone.* I put my head down and kick harder. Moments later a flash of light catches my face. I spin around, shocked, and there's Andrew. He is waving. It takes me a second to realise I've been chasing the wrong dive group.

Giving him the *OK* with my torch – a wobbly circle of light – I trail Andrew back to Liv, and the three of us drift from the open sand towards a nearby reef. With human company in clear view, the dive starts to lose its edge. My panic must have plateaued. Or perhaps it has more to do with me being back inside the cinema of my mask: spectator, not participant.

Fish hover and sleep around us. Bulbous eyes gleam in the torch light. I hope I'm not blinding them. Slinking through the dark water, I note that I no longer feel in charge of my own direction. I am merely hitching a lift on Andrew's current. *Roll up, divers, step this way. Look to your left for the mantis shrimp: see its spearing appendages; those keen eyes watching the phases of the moon. And don't miss the nudibranch on our right – it's a flabellina. Bright colours, frilly edges; looks like a shawl, folks, doesn't it?*

There appear to be no sharks in this bay. No whales or dolphins either. Nothing big, in fact. When we emerge from the water intact, I drag off my wetsuit before I am tied to a rail, and head upstairs to identify what we did see, a routine we've been encouraged to take up by our diving crew. It may not have been the intended effect, but doing this seems to normalise what just happened. *Yes, there's the picture, just how we expected.* I'm reminded of the *i-SPY Nature* book I used to read in the car when I was little. Spy the holly bush, tick the box. Spy the ladybird, tick the box. Spy the dragonfly. Spy the mushroom. Spy the ghost pipefish and hermit crab.

I wonder if this is what diving really is: something trainspotters can do when they run out of trains. I thought there would be more peril involved. Perhaps I've got it wrong.

Andrew comes to sit on the opposite side of the table, raking his damp fringe with puckered fingers.

'So,' he says. 'Deep-dive training tomorrow. Still want to give it a go? You won't see much of Richelieu if you don't.'

Ah, I think. I'd forgotten that might be happening.

'Sure,' I say.

There's the peril.

6

Deeper, Darker

'In limited visibility, it's more difficult to stay with your
buddy and to keep track of where you are and where you're
going. You may feel disorientated when you can't see the
surface or the bottom.'

VISIBILITY,

PADI OPEN WATER MANUAL, 1999–2007

Water does strange things to distance. On land, the idea
of travelling 30 metres sounds harmless. There are
30 metres between my home in London and the main road.
There are 30 metres between the door of Granny Codd's
nursing home and the park. On a zig-zag path like the ones
at Poole beach I could probably climb 30 metres without
many problems. Maybe even push Granny up there in her
wheelchair if she would let me. ('Why don't *you* sit in here
for a change.' 'Great idea, Gran, apart from the fact you can't
stand up because you *never do your stretches*.' 'I'll start tomorrow. Come on. Sit on my lap.')

Descend that distance in water, however, and things start
becoming advanced – officially so, if you're on your PADI

training. By the time you reach 30 metres, certain colours are absorbed. The deeper you go, the more these become imperceptible without torchlight. Red goes first. Then orange and yellow. For a while blues and greens take over. Then the light fades altogether. The air density of your body will be quartered. Carefully crack a raw egg at this depth and its insides will hold and float in a pleasing sphere, instead of flailing and sagging like they would do nearer the surface.

Something else can happen at the 30-metre point and below: a significant change in your state of mind. Nitrogen narcosis is caused by the effect of breathing certain gases under pressure. Like altitude sickness, it's impossible to know how susceptible you might be to this narcosis until it hits. What's more, the effects of narcosis on you may change from one dive to the next. And while the cure is simple – go shallower and it will dissipate – some divers are so disrupted by it they can't even do that. Possessed, almost drunk, they're susceptible to mistakes. Errors and odd decisions that, at depth, can have fatal consequences.

At James Deane's dive shop I met a man called Mark who had been on more than two thousand dives to date. Once, he said, he saw a man swim off into the blue alone, and then start to ascend to the boat at a life-threatening speed. 'He was narc'd up to his brain.' Mark rushed over to pull the man back, but he left the water 'up to his knees', dragging Mark with him. If he hadn't held on regardless the man would have died from the pressure change. As it was, the man was fine. It was Mark who contracted the bends, and needed six hours of decompression treatment at a medical facility.

Another of James's customers described his own experiences with narcosis, a phenomenon sometimes also referred to as 'raptures of the deep'. 'I recognise it coming out,' he said. 'A ringing in the ears, like *wob wob wob*.' Sometimes the panic would make him want to bolt up to the surface. Then, when it set in, 'I don't want to go up. My mind starts to stray. It's a spooky sort of thing.'

James told me about someone he knows who offered his regulator to a fish because of a depth-induced stupor. Another diver I spoke to called the sensation 'feeling groovy.' One likened it to the four horsemen of the apocalypse. For many it is a sense of strange detachment and security. For any diver, narcosis is a warning that the plot is being lost.

Of all the deep diving disasters I've heard about lately – and there seem to be so many – some of the most chilling are the ones in which the diver keeps descending. Where there is no reaction, or capability, to return to the surface. I worry that I'll be susceptible. If the thought of a whale shark can pull me on, couldn't the deep pull me down? It strikes me that confronting a phobia is much like standing on the pinnacle of a tall building: from a great height the ground could neither be more compelling, nor more frightful.

Take a step forward. Let go.

On my second visit to his shop, James Deane lent me a book of diving stories. For a while I sat with it in the safety of the bed, trying to come to terms with the thought of swimming with fish of every shape and size, whether they be miniature or massive. I would put on my best impression of an Oxford CBT specialist. 'If all of these divers have lived to tell their tales,' I'd say out loud, 'why can't you?' The thing was, not all of those stories had positive endings. Within this book, alongside the descriptions of carnivorous fish and large mammals, was the story of a well-known British diver, Rob Palmer. On a live-aboard trip to the Red Sea, it stated, Rob, 'a great champion and pioneer of technical diving', pushed himself to go deeper and deeper with tanks of normal air – the ones that I've used in my own shallow dives, not the tried and tested helium mixes which work to keep your body safe at depth.

On his final dive, accompanied by four others, Rob allegedly headed off well below his companions, two of whom stopped their own descent at 107 metres. The book said Rob was 'at great depth, apparently waving them to continue on down'. And that was the last they saw of him. I pictured this lonely man swimming and swimming, all the world darkening around him. And speculated on the shadowy thoughts that kept him swimming on.

I wonder if I too am being led to a point of no return. It's a thought that's only compounded when YouTube's algorithms offer me up a real-life shocker: a video shot on a helmet camera, by a diving instructor who solo-dived a notorious ocean sinkhole in southeast Sinai, the ravishing Blue Hole. Title: 'Fatal diving accident caught on tape: Yuri Lipski'. Yuri Lipski, the instructor in question, was twenty-two years old.

The video starts just below the surface, where it briefly records two other divers swimming, perhaps 15 metres away. The date is 28 April 2000. Floating himself, Yuri tilts the camera to his face, examining it through the water, breathing air from his tank. After checking the lens he adds a red filter. At this point you can still see other divers. You can see sections of reef. The visibility is good. Air bubbles suggest life and human company. But very soon Yuri Lipski will be alone.

For a while he continues to make more checks of his camera, the surface of the water in clear sight. His breathing is steady. But it is this camera, Tarek Omar said afterwards – Omar being the man who retrieved Yuri's body two days after he died, uploading this found video on to the internet as a cautionary tale years later – that may have fatally tipped Yuri's weight against him. Even just a kilo too much could have done it.

Yuri begins to descend. A diver comes into view. It's not clear if this is his buddy, or if Yuri even has one. Whoever it is does not appear on screen again. There are noises that sound like Yuri attempting to inflate his BCD, trying to stop himself freefalling too fast. But still he continues to drop. There is a reef below him. The ocean, blue at first, becomes gradually gloomier. More spurts can be heard as Yuri attempts again to inflate his vest; attempts to regain control. But it makes no difference. At this point he could release his weight belt to help himself back up. Jettison his camera. Risk the bends to reach the surface. None of these things happen. The edge of the reef appears, blurs and passes. Reaching it, grabbing on, might halt his descent. Instead we watch the water grow darker and darker. Sediment rushes past. The pockets of air in his wetsuit must be compressing. Diminishing his buoyancy. Hurrying him on his way. It's almost impossible to tell now how fast Yuri is sinking, but we can hear him breathing more quickly. And then awful, sporadic sounds – choking, a repressed yell – the sound of this man panicking as he tries to fight the deep. Squeaks. Groans. Restricted gulps.

Less than two-and-a-half minutes since we last saw the surface, it is dark and the human world has vanished. Less than the time it took me to turn on my laptop and find this video.

Something bleeps in warning. It's Yuri's dive computer, positioned on his wrist, alarmed to notify him when any pre-set limits are exceeded. Yuri makes another noise, like a scream. He reaches the stony floor of the ocean sinkhole. Here it is murky and dim. The water is tinged with crimson. There is no life in sight except twisted stalks and branches of coral, looking like tree trunks warped by a nuclear blast. Yuri flails his wrist into view in order to check his computer. Even though he has now hit the bottom his depth gauge is still climbing. He has outpaced it. More flashes of its screen show that the digital figures relaying his depth are rising through the eighties. He checks and checks again. His body is constantly moving. The depth reading reaches the nineties, more than three times the uppermost limit of standard recreational diving. Yuri's noises of distress become strained. His helmet camera turns onto its side, uprooting the picture; making the video wonky. He seems to be flailing across the ground, scudding over rocks. A loud whoosh of air escapes. Perhaps this is when his BCD bursts, an event that his retriever, Tarek Omar, noted later in an interview with *Der Spiegel*. For now though the reddened dust is flying. Yuri struggles over the seabed with his final breaths. This may be when he starts fitting, his muscles sent into spasm by a toxic build-up of oxygen. We see a fin. Hear the squeak of rubber. Metal clatters on stone. There is a noise of crunching. Thick clouds of sediment fill the screen. Yuri's breathing is barely there now. The camera stalls with a beep. The picture freezes. But the water behind continues to move with his body. You can hear it. Moments later, we cut to the inside of a room with a tiled floor. It is five days after the video began. 'OK,' says a man, off camera. We see two pairs of legs, sitting down. The film cuts to blue and then ends.

In an interview with the *Observer*, Tarek Omar recounted how Yuri turned his back on the two weeks of site-specific training needed before a dive at the Blue Hole could safely take place. An hour after Yuri met Omar and declined this offer of training, he was sinking to his death. Hundreds of other divers have also died at this site, its clear blue water inviting them down, its rock formations beckoning them on, until they lose their sense of depth as much as of danger. 'They want to get into deep water, before they get into deep knowledge,' said Omar to the *Observer*. Impetuous divers aiming to break their personal bests on holiday; trying to reach landmark depths like 100 metres, for instance, in a place where not all instructors care exactly how much of a novice their customer is. Not when they're being paid a decent sum.

If you don't make mistakes you'll be fine, right? Perhaps that's what some of these deep divers think. Perhaps that's why they're able to keep coming back, even when facing the news that yet more people have died doing what they're planning to do. Perhaps they see themselves as somehow immune.

Perhaps that's how I'll feel if I do enough dives.

One day, while still in London, I contacted Tarek Omar to find out how he felt about his own involvement with diving and the Blue Hole. The man had earned two nicknames in his career: 'Bone Collector' and 'Keeper of Dahab's Divers' Cemetery' – that cemetery being the Blue Hole dive site itself. I'd read that Tarek had retrieved more bodies at the Blue Hole than he could count. And all pro bono. He had risked his own life to bring back the corpses of people confused by the water, mistaking eerie lights for the surface, pushing themselves past boundaries they didn't understand, making minor mistakes that, at those depths, turned catastrophic. I read that, to find the bodies, Tarek would calculate the point where they had reached the bottom, then 'allow his body to drift, as if he too were dead.' Some people would call that tempting fate. I wanted to know what Tarek would call it. I looked him up on Facebook and sent a message.

Tarek agreed to reply to my questions by email, so I sent them over. In the days I waited to hear from him, I imagined him being torn away from his screen and summoned back into the water. Strapping the next body to himself, perhaps – one report I found stated that they average one a month – and sending it up to the surface. Why, I asked, did he think the Blue Hole was the site of so many fatalities?

'Ego and attitude,' came Tarek's reply in due course. 'Ignorance, lack of deep-water knowledge, lack of training.'

I had heard it said that many visitors to Dahab see the site's conditions and feel safe: the warmth, the low current, the high visibility. That is a fatal error in a place you don't know well. Tarek, on the other hand, has dived there for almost thirty years. In one interview he likened the site to his garden. In an another it was his living room. There are bones at the bottom of that living room. Divers buried at the end of that garden. But, he insisted in his email to me, 'the site is safe and I am the living proof.' More than that: diving there makes Tarek happy. 'I was the first to fully explore the Blue Hole and with my knowledge and experience of it I have been helpful to others.' He added, 'I feel connected to it spiritually.'

Tarek told me that he found life out of the water riskier than life in it. 'Underwater life is clear,' he wrote, 'then you can take all safety measures.' Out of the water, he said, the risks were more plentiful, and harder to identify. In one article I read, Tarek said that he finds watching horror films more frightening than diving in the Blue Hole. Then he stopped himself. 'The ocean squeezes you, you can actually hear it if you go in a submarine. It sounds romantic but it's actually very dangerous.'

Unlike the other divers I'd spoken to, Tarek – perhaps unsurprisingly, given his Blue Hole experiences – was unafraid to make clear links between death and his passion. He wrote, 'I started diving in 1996 in Sinai after two of my friends died in the water while diving. It gave me the reason to understand why they died and also it was the best thing to do living near the Red Sea.' He continued, 'later I started to be fascinated by depth and to accept the risks associated with mixed gas extreme deep diving.' But despite accepting these risks, when I asked Tarek if he thought diving was dangerous, his reply to me was plain. 'Not really if you know what you are doing and if you're balancing your ability, your fitness mentally and physically, and not exceeding physiological limits.'

Tarek told me he had seen Yuri Lipski's video on numerous occasions, playing it as a teaching aid to highlight the hazards to divers. I asked him what he thought about when he watched it. 'What goes in my mind is he died doing what he loves to do,' he replied. 'Sometimes I think what if it was me – what I can do to overcome such underwater situation.'

'Why exactly did Yuri die?' I asked.

'Firstly because he didn't keep a handle on what he was capable of,' Tarek replied. 'Secondly I believe in God and I know that everyone has their time to die and this was Yuri's time . . . Sad,' he wrote, 'but it is a fact.'

And so we came back to spirituality. Seeing so much death at the Blue Hole, said Tarek, makes him feel both sad and stressed. But also, he wrote, it 'gets me closer to God.' I try entertaining the thought that searching for whale sharks could be my spiritual journey. Framing it in that way seems nuts, at first. The whale shark isn't something I want to worship.

But maybe there is something to this. A sense of surrender I'm craving, or something more tangible. Perhaps the ocean is my higher power. Like a god it can remove me from myself. It takes and it gives. Plus any attempts to subdue it are always guaranteed to fail.

If the ocean was God, what would that make the whale shark? A miracle, maybe. A prophet. I wish I knew. I wish, as it does for Tarek, the world underwater would make things clearer for me.

I was still thinking about Yuri Lipski, about sinking further down into the dark, when I talked to Vicky, a woman who has been diving since she was twelve. Vicky has learnt how to weld underwater. She teaches diving regularly, and acts as a safety monitor for companies wanting to film beneath the waves. She also works at the London Diving Chamber, a medical unit where divers go to be treated for the bends. Even she has struggled with the deep. 'I felt out of my depth,' Vicky said, referring to her first and only dive to 100 metres. For a moment she laughed sarcastically at her own joke. Then she grew serious and stared at the ceiling, remembering.

'That was scary. You've got two tanks on your back and three tanks on your front, you're checking your computers, you've never been there before. There's so much crush depth you've got no buoyancy. You're filling your BCD with air and you're trying to come off 100 metres, trying to get up by kicking. But it's difficult to swim down there and I've got no air and I'm putting air in, I'm putting air in, and I take one breath in and I see my gas going down and I'm thinking, *I can't get up, I can't get up.* My friend comes down and is like, *Get up!* and I'm like *Yeah, doofus. I know.* Because even a minute at extra depth is going to affect your decompression schedule. There was a moment of, *What if I can never get up again?* Which is totally irrational because down there you're 100 per cent task-focused. You're staring at your gauges, you know your time schedule, you've got everything written down, you know where you're meant to be at what depth, and you've just got to go with it . . . '

I imagine being overwhelmed by water. Being held down. Kicking against it with all that I have, unable to rise, going nowhere. The word *terrible* barely covers it. *Atrocious. Appalling. Hideous.*

Vicky describes it a different way. 'It was so exciting,' she says.

My mouth hangs open. The grin spreads across her face.

*

It is risk, not excitement, that's on my mind as I finish the PADI chapter I need to read to prepare for my first advanced deep dive. In the morning, as I kit up to enter the water, Andrew casually mentions that, if we're lucky, we'll come across the whitetip shark that usually patrols this particular area. As if I needed more excuses to worry.

I am fully prepared for the worst. To lose myself in the blue. But we enter the water and 30 metres looks just like a dimmer version of what it is at 18. Moreover, Andrew has chosen a spot without a deep drop, so there's no chance of me falling indefinitely to a pressurised death like Yuri Lipski. Instead I rest on my knees beside him as he points, almost *Blue Peter*-like, at a laminated colour chart on which all the squares have turned cobalt, then cracks an egg to demonstrate the pressure's holding effect on its insides. Immediately, accidentally, he pierces the yolk and the whole lot leaks away, destroying the hovering sphere, ruining the trick. I glance about me, watching for sharks, but none appear in my eyeline. Nor do I experience any moods that feel like what I've heard about narcosis.

We stay that low for only a matter of minutes, then ascend to shallower water. The rest of the dive is tranquil: another giant moray that doesn't care; a peculiar yellow boxfish with a cuboid body and leopard-like spots; a couple of fish known as seamoths (camouflaged bottom-dwellers with fanned fins); plus a unicornfish with a profile like Alfred Hitchcock. Long nose, tight lips, large chin.

Afterwards, stepping on to the boat, I shed my kit and gorge on the limitless air. I stretch my arms. I feel light. I feel unconstricted. This is relief, but I know it won't last. Later we will dive in search of giant manta rays, then continue on our journey. Back down into the water we will go; ever closer to what awaits at Richelieu.

7

To Richelieu and Beyond

'As a diver you'll swim with new and fascinating underwater organisms. Some will swim up to you curiously, while others will flee your presence.'

THE DIVE ENVIRONMENT,
PADI OPEN WATER MANUAL, 1999–2007

One day before we reach Richelieu Rock, Andrew and I ascend from the underwater valley of Koh Bon. We've counted endless parrotfish. Eyeballed a part-hidden octopus. The sights we passed were picturesque and quirky. But the vast arena of Koh Bon seemed to lack something. Something large enough to fill it. Moments later, Liv and her instructor, Kwan, appear at the surface a few metres away.

'Did you see?' shouts Liv, eyes shining through her mask.

Please not the whale shark.

I take a deep breath. 'See what?' I shout back.

'The giant *manta*!' she sings.

Back on the boat, all the divers are buzzing about what they've just witnessed: a giant ray with a 4-metre wingspan. It circled the rock and flew over a diver. I watch Liv's video of it. The creature looks fictitious, built like a villain from *Zelda*, with a white semi-skeletal stomach, and two horn-shaped protuberances standing guard either side of its open mouth. Andrew and I are silent.

Koh Bon is the home of the giant manta. We'll dive it again before dinner. We'll meet this fish with its beastly wingspan and then I can test how I cope.

We dive again before dinner.

We do not see the giant manta.

I worry I've been cursed. Or that Andrew has been cursed, and I've been caught up in his curse by association. Whatever is happening, I fear it does not bode well for whale sharks at Richelieu Rock. Neither does what Kwan – Liv's instructor – has been telling us lately. After almost every dive now, he says we should have come to the Andaman seven years ago. That, back then, there were giant sea creatures everywhere. Everywhere a manta. Everywhere a massive shark. Maybe even a whale.

'Four metres is nothing,' he says. 'Seven years ago you get 7 metres manta.' The way he tells it, the sea around here is becoming a no-go for big fish. They've mostly disappeared. Not disappeared. Been killed.

The evidence is all around us; signs showing that man is the greatest threat around here. At night, while we make our way to our dive sites for the following day, spotlights burn across the horizon. They signify night fishermen, scouring the water for anything they can sell. The thought of whatever's beneath them being hauled up is not something I want to contemplate, but still I imagine these weird creatures suffocating. Their guts shoot out of gaping mouths, ripped from their bodies by pressure. I can almost smell the blood smearing the decks. I wonder how many of these fishermen have wrapped their nets around a giant manta. Around a whale shark. And what it felt like to haul that catch back to shore. I wonder whether it would have been a triumph for these men – or whether it could also have felt like a tragedy.

I feel a deep disgust. Especially at myself. Because even in spite of these killings – what I hear, and what I imagine – I am still repulsed by the victims of this industry; by the fish themselves. As I sit in my cabin, unable to relax, these conflicted feelings transport me back to my mother's garden, where we dug a small pond in the lawn when I was eight. I remember how, for more than a decade, the pond was a home for goldfish, newts and frogs. But one spring, during a break from university, when my issues with fish had already been firmly established, something about the pond changed.

It started with dead toads. There were so many. At first we thought a neighbour's cat had killed them, but we could not find any bite marks or signs of blood. The night before their bodies appeared, I'd looked out of my bedroom window to see the pond water thrashing with life: the toads were mating there as they did every year. But this time, for the first time, they did not leave the pond when they were done. They died in it. And, for reasons that have always stayed a mystery, they continued to die in it, jumping into the water to mate, never coming out. We fished out their elastic bodies for days, retrieving distended pink bellies and gluey eyes. We put stones in the water to help any last stragglers climb to the edge. After a while the bodies stopped appearing. We were relieved.

The following week, I walked to the lawn to hang my clean clothes out to dry. My mother was working, so I was on my own. As I pegged up a towel, a movement in the pond caught my attention. I looked across to see a goldfish on the surface, belly up. I dropped the towel and hurried over. The fish was twitching. Two other goldfish were dead beside it. Another was fruitlessly trying to swim on its side.

The vision was grotesque. These fish were clearly dying and needed help. But the look of them was so frightening that I did not know how I could help them. Another fish floated up from the gloom and started rolling over. I urged Mum to come through the front door and save us, but knew that the timing was wrong. It wouldn't happen. *I could do this if I wasn't me*, I thought. *Maybe I can play mother. Hold myself in.*

Panicking, I ran to the outside tap, filled up buckets with water, found the net Mum used to pull out fallen leaves, and aimed to retrieve the few creatures still showing signs of life. My movements were clumsy. I felt like I was doing more harm than good, distressing the fish with my motions; pushing them into the weeds instead of scooping them cleanly up. I knew that if I didn't calm down I would kill them all the quicker.

Had Granny Codd been around at that point she would no doubt have said, 'They're more afraid of you, Georgina.' But she wasn't there, she was somewhere else – I didn't know where – Marks and Spencer's, maybe, like all good grannies – and anyway, her comment wouldn't have made me less scared or revolted. Arms trembling, I transferred a couple of live goldfish into a bucket apiece, then, too late, considered that the shock of this cold, just-poured water might finish them off. Indeed, as I watched in horror, this was exactly what seemed to be happening: on reaching the bucket, each fish gave a spurt of movement, finally righting itself, then quickly stopping, becoming less responsive than before. Rocking the buckets back and forth, I tried to wash their gills through with fresh oxygen. But even this animated them only temporarily.

I turned away from the bucket-fish, lost causes both, and

went back to the pond. Another sick fish was now surfacing. In the midst of my probing to catch it, one of the floating dead creatures near it moved. This Lazarus fluttered its tail but went nowhere, like a wind-up toy that's been knocked to the ground. Perhaps, I thought, all the dead-looking fish were alive. With a dreadful sense of responsibility – a responsibility I never wanted – I sank the net beneath them and carried them through the air towards a third bucket.

Almost as soon as these creatures met clean water, their movements stopped. Dead fish, dead fish. Dead. All around me bodies lay, two of them horribly gasping, most of them horribly still. I sat on the patio stones, fixed by several sets of accusing eyes. By the time Mum came home, only one fish from the pond was still alive. She gave it to the neighbours. We didn't deserve to keep it. Toads had polluted the water and we hadn't made it right.

That summer the pond turned a urinous yellow, with a density of sediment that was impossible to see through. Nothing lived inside it. Land snails fell in and died, their fleshy feet softening upside-down until they dissolved, increasing the pond's toxicity even more. I asked Mum when she was going to clean the water. She said she wasn't sure, that it was too hard a job to think about. I thought about clearing it out myself, then thought about the bodies at the bottom, putrefying. Eventually I stopped asking Mum. And stopped looking out of the window. There was no life to watch there anyway.

Three nights I've been on this liveaboard now. In the early hours we moor at Richelieu Rock, Thailand's number one diving destination. Richelieu, the site of my dreams and anxieties. As the sun rises over the waves I lean back on my elbows and fail to keep my mind calm. Instead I get trapped in the weeds of my brain, and spend energy trying to summon and send off what's coming. *Just turn up, will you, not too close, and then I can hide behind somebody else, but actually don't turn up because I'm not really sure I'm ready.* It's exactly like the time I went in with the dolphins just a fortnight ago – exhausting fluctuations between terror and excitement. In some ways I seem to have come so far since then, so quickly. In other ways, I don't feel like I've made much progress at all. I think of the number of fish I've seen since leaving Alex and New Zealand. Each one I've logged is a fish I no longer need to be afraid of meeting. I've shared the water with them and survived.

Only, every specimen I've logged so far has been nothing compared to the whale shark. Even the giant morays were smaller than me. Longer, yes, but still a fish that, theoretically, I could wrestle into submission. The big things, though – the ones that won't fit under my arm – I still don't know what I'll do if they turn against me. And that is alarming.

Perhaps I could swim away. Perhaps that's the answer. Could I swim faster than a whale shark? I wonder how fast they go. I flick through my notes and read up on it. The majority of sources say it's a fairly constant 3 miles per hour at the surface, which is not good news for me: there's no way I can swim at that speed for long.

Perhaps I should swim *at* the whale shark if things go wrong. Perhaps not.

Years back, on my first and only visit to Canada, my cousin and had a similar dilemma. If we were to see a grizzly bear should we run towards it, or run away? Neither my cousin nor I could remember. For most of the trip we thought it was run away. But no. Turns out neither option was quite right. Grizzly bears can reach high speeds. They chase cars and climb trees and have claws like knives. They also don't appreciate being threatened. Instead stand your ground, say the experts.

Avoid making eye contact then slowly back away. If the bear still decides to go for you, make yourself big and act like you might be dangerous. Just pray it doesn't see through your ruse, because as soon as it does you're going to get a scalping.

Shark speculations hang heavy on my nerves. I feel like my heart is on the starting block, gearing up for full pelt. I need to breathe deeply before I get carried away – more carried away than I already am, that is.

The next air tank ought to do it. During my research on CBT skills, I've learned that breathing slowly soothes all manner of brain problems. Handily, that's what scuba makes you do. I try it now, pretending I'm on oxygen and, as I inhale, a well-meaning rational voice in my head makes its presence felt, very quietly. It's saying that whale sharks, unlikely grizzly bears, can't scalp me.

Ah, I think back in reply. *But what about Jacques Cousteau's American friend? The one who was 'seriously hurt' when his arm was caught in a whale shark's mouth; who 'suffered extensive bruises and lost considerable portions of his skin'. Is that not, in effect, a scalping of the arm?*

The well-meaning rational voice in my head falls silent. It seems to be pondering the point. After several seconds of peace it clears its throat. I pause in my breathing exercises, patiently waiting to hear the next piece of advice.

DO NOT PUT YOUR ARM IN A WHALE SHARK'S MOUTH, shrieks the voice.

Yes, my rational friend. I think we can all agree that's a wise course of action.

We will dive four times at Richelieu Rock today, following in the footsteps (or fin kicks) of Jacques-Yves Cousteau himself. It is alleged that Cousteau was the first to discover this world-famous site in 1989, thanks to tip-offs from local

fishermen, and that he named it for the robe-like draping of
sea life across the rock, a sight said to be reminiscent of the
seventeenth-century garb of Cardinal Richelieu. Others say
the British Royal Navy knew about this spot first and named
the submerged rock after a general. Either way, Cousteau was
the one who made Richelieu big. He's the reason we're all
poised at this place right now, and most likely in more ways
than one. I try to imagine how many of us assembled here
took up diving because of Cousteau. Certainly, we are all
using the modern descendant of his Aqualung (the first piece
of kit for breathing underwater that was both self-contained
and open-circuit – i.e. expelling the used air instead of recy-
cling it). And when I say 'us assembled here', I don't only
mean our boat of computer-fluent Spaniards. As I emerge
from my cabin and head to the deck, I see many vessels
moored around this rock: five, six – possibly more on their
way. All are liveaboards piled high with divers. All want to
share the same currents, see the same things. No doubt most
will be hoping to find whale sharks.

By merely observing the surface, you'd never know the
attraction of this site. From time to time, the waves part to
reveal the rock's highest point – a small assortment of stubby
crags, poking through the water. It looks like nothing; a
captain's hazard, no more. Yet here lies the Holy Grail of the
Thai diving industry.

As we kit up, my back curves into a familiar position,
ready to receive the heavy tank. My shoulder muscles groan.
This is it, chaps, I tell my sinewy friends. *This is the dive we've
been waiting for. This is what the whole lot's been about. Get this
right and we'll never need to do this nonsense again.* It's just as
well. Buying my place on this liveaboard trip means my Ted
travels will already be too tight for comfort. There's no extra
money to spare.

Liv and I complete our checks. We lurch away from the crew's tiring game of tying-zips-together. And then we're jumping in.

As our dive group descends, it's immediately clear why the world makes a beeline for Richelieu. Not only is it large and covered with life, it's astoundingly, richly exquisite. Indigo fronds of soft coral crawl with fish, crustaceans and molluscs. There are so many different species here I lose count. We are tourists in a bustling city of colour. Lionfish, porcupine-fish, boxfish, frogfish, pipehorses, boxer shrimps, dancing shrimps, tiger cowries, batfish, barracuda, potato groupers, trevallies, scorpionfish, yellow snapper, hermit crabs. Zebra morays with their black and white stripes. These are just the creatures I can identify from reading our liveaboard's limited book collection. At one point Kwan lifts up a cleaner shrimp, lowers it into his open mouth, and lets the decapod work on extracting miniscule pieces of food from his teeth. It's gross. And mesmerising. Later, Andrew passes one to me and I watch transfixed, almost paralysed, as its spindly mass picks delicately away to clear the dirt beneath my fingernails. Job done, the shrimp scuttles back on to its ledge. I'm more than 20 metres underwater, and a shrimp has given me a manicure. As if that's normal. As if I should have expected it. The place is unreal. And, as we move away from the world's weirdest beauty salon, I am suddenly struck by the effect of ten days of diver training: I just let a shrimp do my nails. *An actual shrimp.* What's more, it did my nails to perfection.

Every minute or so I tear myself away from the enthralling sights of the rock, its harmonious collage of species, and look up to the surface, or out to the blue. I wonder where the whale shark is. Have I missed it or is it coming? Then my attention is diverted back to the creatures before me, an arm's length away, sometimes less. I'm still breathing slowly.

I'm still with my group. I think I feel, I *do* feel, surprisingly safe. Able, fit and not exceeding my limits.

When we turn a corner, we find ourselves facing a trail of hanging divers, suspended in a line from the rock, tailing back. The underwater city has an underwater traffic jam; an intrusion that mars all sense of beauty and balance. I recoil at the sight – then realise that I, too, am an invader, potentially disrupting what I thought I was just passing through. My mind starts whirring. At the same time, to my relief, my group moves off. *We're not the same kind of people as the queuers,* I tell myself, desperate to justify my place in this scene. *My dive group knows the importance of flow. It knows not to intrude. It knows when to keep moving.*

This is a game of semantics. I know it's a game of semantics. But for the moment, at least, it works. The pang of guilt eases.

As I follow the others around the side we cast a glance at the subject of the first queue diver's camera shot: a couple of tigertail seahorses on a rock, small and Crayola-yellow. Satisfied, our group edges away, while the other divers wait to snap their identical seahorse pictures. A minute later, I look back around and see an incident flaring up. Kwan and the man from the front of the queue are squaring up to each other with violent gestures. It looks as if they're about to fight, but after some chest-puffery and menacing finger points, the two of them pull apart without throwing a punch. Later I learn that the man objected to Liv snapping her own quick seahorse photo. He considered it jumping the line. Then Kwan objected to that. Goodness knows what the seahorses thought of it all. Goodness knows what they think every day, when neoprene creatures float over their home and track each movement they make through massive lenses.

Sixty-four minutes later, I emerge from this first dive and, despite the lack of whale sharks, I am exhilarated. We've had one attempt down on one section of rock, with three dives left to scale as much of the rest as we can before leaving. In other words, the whale sharks have time to appear. I've done my planning, after all. Picked the right time of year. Completed the right training. Put myself in exactly the right location. All I need do now is wait and stay calm; remember to breathe.

So I wait.

And I wait.

And I wait.

Dive Two and Dive Three: no whale sharks. Nudibranchs, coral groupers, more morays. A flatworm like the pelt of a Pokémon, spiked brown with orange flecks. But no whale sharks.

Come on, Dive Four. Come on. This will be my last dive at Richelieu Rock. I suit myself up. I fidget on the deck. I cast my wishes out to sea. I dive.

And would you believe it? That whale shark, the one that's been circling inside my head for months, the one I've travelled for many days and 7500 miles to see –

Well –

It doesn't show up.

8

A Void

'Divers who have a problem and panic lose self control . . .
Sudden, unreasoned fear and instinctive inappropriate
actions replace controlled, appropriate actions.'

PROBLEM MANAGEMENT,
PADI OPEN WATER MANUAL, 1999–2007

I have lost control. Of my goal. Of my sense of purpose.
This was not supposed to happen.

It is happening.

Everything should have been wrapped up by now, but it
isn't. After two weeks of inland travels with Ted, occupying
ourselves with water fights and *som tum* salads and temples,
we're back home where we started, the excitement has
worn off and I feel anxious again. I may have gained a few
stories for Granny, but essentially I've conquered nothing.
I'm feeling the need for a focal point but there aren't any
whale sharks nearby. It's not like I have indefinite funds to
keep looking.

Should I have a job? I should probably have a job. That's
right. I'm supposed to be going to Bristol and finding a job.

After a few days back in London, nesting, resting, catching up on sleep, I try to embark on the next phase of the plan as if the last went perfectly well. It's time to make my way down to the West Country. Ted will follow soon, and our goodbye is loving, filled with hugs.

'Bristol together!'

'Tedgie for ever!'

Perhaps this is my focal point. Perhaps I don't need whale sharks after all.

En route to my next destination, I stop for a weekend with Mum and Granny Codd. They're both excited to see me, neither one bothered about my sharking failures.

'Never mind,' says Mum, at the train station.

'Never mind,' says Granny Codd later. At the nursing home, over a cup of tea, I tell her about the things I've swum with over the past few weeks: the urchins, the eels, the fish. My brief encounter with dolphins.

'Did you *really?*' she exclaims. 'Well, well, well.'

'I wrote it all down,' I tell her. 'But there's some prostitute stuff in there which I probably need to cut for your sensitive eyes.'

Granny Codd grins and wrinkles her nose. Then she reaches for her tea cup. I notice how much effort the movement takes her, and move the handle towards her outstretched fingers. After a shaky sip, she turns and looks out of the window.

'Oh!' she cries after a moment. 'The animal!'

'What animal?' I ask.

She turns back to me, eyes wide and full of delight. 'I don't know. It's brown. Lots of – Hmm. Very sweet and soft. Can you see? Is it there?'

I stand up and peer through the window. I can see branches

and leaves. The road past the park. 'Brown, sweet and soft, you say?'

'Yes,' says Granny, beaming.

'I think it must've gone.'

'Oh.'

'Must have been a fast one,' I add. 'A squirrel?'

'No,' she says, with certainty. Then she looks at me again, and instantly her face is pure confusion. 'Was it?'

'Probably a squirrel,' I say brightly, trying to mask my concern. 'Brown and soft. Fits the bill.'

'OK,' she giggles. 'It smiles, almost. It's very sweet and funny.'

I'd wanted to ask Granny about her poems. About the purple man in the boat. About her lost first husband. But today is not the day.

It takes a while for my job-hunt to lead anywhere. In the meantime, I stay on a small farm outside Bristol, exchanging room and board for a few hours of work, sometimes mowing the grass, sometimes picking the rhubarb, sometimes clearing the nettles, or pruning the orchard, or ironing the sheets. My weeks of travelling have awakened a new desire to stay out in the open. And the constant tasks stop me from thinking too much about what I have missed – and what I am still missing.

One day, during a tea break in the garden, I learn that I've been called back for a second interview at a solicitors' office in the lovely, leafy locale of Queen Square. I'm pleased. I want this job. It's a decent salary, interesting work and a step up from what I was doing before in London. The interview goes well. When I leave the office, the hirers are laughing with me and not at me. The four of us are all laughing *together*. I'm fairly sure that's a good sign, so when I arrive back at the farm, I call Ted.

'Do you want to come down and look for our new home this weekend?' I ask.

'Oh,' replies Ted. 'Er . . . ' He hesitates.

I wait.

'Maybe not this weekend,' he says, eventually. 'I'm kinda busy this weekend. Maybe another weekend?'

Except, it turns out, that's not what Ted means at all. What he means, he admits when pressed, is possibly 'no weekend ever'. At some point over the past month, he's not sure when exactly, he's decided he doesn't want to move to Bristol. Never mind the multiple visits we made here, scoping out various neighbourhoods to live in. Never mind what we've been saying to friends and family about *the next stage of our lives*. He wants to stay in London, Ted thinks, where his mates are. In fact, he wants us – him, me, his mates – to all move in together. And this is the first I've heard of it.

Afterwards, a week later than promised, the solicitors from Queen Square send me an email. I haven't got the job. 'Thank you once again for the interest and commitment you have demonstrated to this exercise.'

Exercise. Apparently that was an exercise.

I say goodbye to the picturesque farm with the gorgeous trees and orderly tasks, and slump back to the capital with my bags. I can't keep this up. Ted and I have things to address. Bristol must go on hold. And now I am back where I started again, back in the city I thought I'd left, not only thoroughly jobless but suddenly insecure, living with a man I love but potentially can't depend on.

'I can't believe you've done this,' I say, shoving my farm clothes into the washing basket. 'Bristol was so NICE.'

'It wasn't for me, though,' says Ted, putting down his book on the bedside table. 'We don't know anyone there.'

'We know each other. And we could make new friends.'

'I wouldn't have been happy.'

'Well, I'm not happy here!' I shout. Then I collapse on the bed beside him. Study my fingers. 'Sorry,' I say. 'Both of us ought to be happy. It's . . . it's probably a good thing that you changed your mind about Bristol.'

'Thanks.'

I sigh. 'Note: I only said "probably".'

London feels oppressively familiar. It feels like all I'm doing here is treading filthy water. I want to feel something other than frustration. I want meaning. And, although Ted and I talk at length about what we should do next, neither of us seem able to find a solution that feels right.

Framed against all that's now happening, the idea of searching for whale sharks is less daunting than ever before. It seems so certain. So concrete. Such a clear and measurable way for my life to move forward. Which is a shame because I'm broke, and can't keep looking until I've earned more money. Together, Ted and I form a compromise: after two weeks of stasis and pondering, we decide I should take another break from London instead of rushing to bag my next place of employment. He thinks it's important I work out exactly what *I* want from our life after almost six years as a couple. The truth is, I'm sure I know what that is already: I want, while I'm away, for Ted to change his mind about staying in London. I want him to decide to move to Bristol. To pick me over his friends.

I am going to play the waiting game – and this is what I tell him. Ted smiles. Shakes his head.

'Oh, Gogs,' he says, in his *what-can-I-do-with-you* voice.

I plan my escape to a random town in Shropshire, where a lesbian couple, advertising online, say they'd like to exchange room and board for four hours of gardening a day, maybe some cooking too, here and there. The offer sounds good to me. I have no better thoughts on how to stay occupied and fed during this period of limbo. Ted is being supportive. Perhaps he is hoping that I'll finally get the wanderlust out of my system. That I will relent and decide to stay in London after all. I know what I think about that.

'We could end up in Shropshire,' I suggest, assembling a bag for the third time in three months. 'That might be a step forward.'

'Shropshire? You're insane,' he counteracts.

'You're insane. Why would I want to squeeze into a house with a load of your friends?'

'It'd be fun.'

'I've lived in houses of five before. The word "fun" does not spring to mind.'

I arrive in Shropshire in summer, and immediately note that the garden, my charge, is the size of about two parking spaces. Like many parking spaces, it is also almost entirely paved over. This is not what I pictured when I pictured myself gardening.

I quickly learn that the work these women want me to do – let's call them Luna and Sunshine – consists of a random assortment of things, including:

- Brushing cobwebs off bins
- Scraping microscopic sprouts from paving stones
- Sweeping specks of dirt off flowerpots and ironwork
- Re-varnishing a table and four chairs
- Editing Sunshine's memoirs
- Digging a flat trench in the dirt – *perfectly* flat – 'Here's the spirit level, Georgie' – then filling this perfectly flattened trench with gravel (a substance that couldn't be less flat if a steamroller rode over it).

The agreement was that I would stay here for two months in total, living in an uninsulated shed that the ladies loftily refer to as 'The Summer Pavilion'. On the plus side, at least I don't have to share this draughty space with three friends of Ted's I barely know.

From the outset it seems highly unlikely that I'll make it to two months. But morbid fascination keeps me gripped in Luna and Sunshine's clutches. One of their dogs, for instance, has two rows of perfectly formed lower teeth, one neatly lined up behind the other. It's baffling. He looks like a North Atlantic Sheepshead, a fish with multiple rows of teeth of its own. I cannot help but stare.

The domestic arrangements are similarly compelling. The door to the bathroom, for example, is made of unfrosted glass, and comes off the only passageway connecting all the rooms. This means that when anyone's inside the bathroom – showering, perhaps, or perched on the toilet – there's nowhere for them to hide. I'm instructed to announce my intentions, so that neither Luna nor Sunshine will walk past and see me in action.

At breakfast, which I eat alone – the ladies seem to prefer whichever side of the house I'm not in – I read the latest issue of *The Mountain Astrologer* (sample feature: 'The Astrology of Pop'). When not in the garden I write, walk the dogs, wash up, learn to make Sunshine's Special Coffee™, and practise cleaning the shower in just the right way, a trick that involves the careful configuration of a houseplant and a chair.

Often, when I'm sat on my own, preparing for my next session of cobweb clearance, I hear Sunshine screaming at Luna from their bedroom. Sunshine can barely walk, and takes out her frustration in shrill and sporadic ways. At the slightest provocation she behaves like an overgrown baby. When I serve her a dish of pasta for dinner one evening, she starts to panic.

'What is this?' she puffs. 'It's a funny colour.' She turns to Luna. 'I don't know what it is. Luna? What is it?'

I tell her it's what we talked about last night, what she said she'd like to try for her next dinner: florets of fried cauliflower in a creamy tomato sauce, served up with pasta and parmesan.

Sunshine pulls a face. 'It looks like *salmon*,' she says.

After we've got to know each other better, Luna and Sunshine offer to give me a tarot reading. I readily accept. I'd like to know what might be around the corner, what Ted and I will end up doing, for instance, and whether I'll ever find myself a whale shark. With the help of computer software that apparently cost them more than £1200, my hosts plot out my charts, reporting everything they see. First they tell me I am 'very Capricorn', which makes sense, I guess, since Capricorn is my star sign. Next, they tell me that I have 'shit in my eyes'. For a moment I wonder if this is a term of endearment exclusive to Shropshire, but clearly not: they go on to tell me I'm in a phase of selfishness; that I should help others more. In a less pointed tone, they add that something about Pluto makes me attracted to murkiness and depths. And that, in spring, something major is going to go down in my life. We round off with the report that there is a storm in my personality. And that I have 'learning development problems'. I thank them, wash up, and return to the shed, reflecting that our relationship may not be quite as congenial as I thought. It's not like I thought it was hugely congenial to begin with.

Weeks later, in fact, I'll discover, through a process of mutual write-ups on the website that brought us together, that I'd made an unfavourable impression on Luna and Sunshine from the start. I'll read that I was not what they had been hoping for; that, despite my best efforts to make this work, they saw me as inflexible and false. I'll read that they thought that I was crap at cooking, and – more damningly still – that the way I fussed over their dogs wasn't *nearly* effusive enough. I'll marvel at how we managed to find so many negative attributes in each other. But, until then, when I try to extract their opinions of me – to learn how they think I'm doing – I'll be met with a pair of smiles; a pause, and then praise.

On the phone, Ted asks when I'm going to come back to London. He suspects that my stay in Shropshire will end badly. I've been thinking the same thing myself, more with every day I spend as a live-in helper, but I want to see *how* it ends badly.

'The set-up sounds crazy,' he says.

'It is crazy,' I agree. But still I don't leave. It dawns on me that seeing this car crash through has become my temporary purpose. And for now this purpose is more achievable than chasing the great unknown of great-sized sharks, not to mention the great unknown that is becoming Ted and me.

Mum, too, suggests I leave when she calls for a morning catch-up.

'And do what?' I reply.

'You could move in with me for a while.'

'I'm not sure that'd be great for me and Ted.'

'Maybe not,' says Mum. 'Just a thought.' She changes the subject. On Sunday it's Granny Codd's ninety-eighth birthday. There's a family tea to plan. A wheelchair taxi to book. At the end of the week, with Luna and Sunshine's approval, I take off for a few days, and head down to Poole.

Granny is tired. As the party starts she wears her politest smile. Gradually she turns irritable. Her hearing aids aren't working. Her lower back is sore.

'Can I go home?' she asks me about an hour in. But it's Sunday and the wheelchair taxi man has a full afternoon.

My cousins and I take it in turns to sit with her, away from the table of food. Granny isn't hungry. She isn't in the mood. Josie – the aunt who once persuaded my uncle to climb up a water butt – rings around and manages to bring forward the ride to the nursing home. When the cab comes I help Granny in, and sit down to travel back with her.

'Sorry you're feeling rotten,' I say. 'What do you think you'll do for the rest of the day?'

'Lie down,' she says, with an effort at laughing. Before the engine starts, her eyes are closed. The next day, as I head up north, I'm updated with a text message from Mum: *Granny is still tired, but seems much perkier.*

Sometimes, when I stop to wonder exactly what I am doing, I dwell on the feeling of purpose I had in Thailand. Get up, dive, eat, dive, rest, dive, eat, then try to sleep, testing my limits a little with every descent, all the while approaching a significant – hopefully, positive – conclusion.

Every day I find I crave that purpose more. I wish I had that positive conclusion.

Back with the ladies, I daydream about a time when I can book flights and shark-search again. The more I research, the more I realise how naïve I was to think I'd find a whale shark on my first diving adventure, never mind feel totally ready to swim with one. It turns out that, even once I've sorted things with Ted, then amassed more funds to travel back over the oceans, locating a whale shark is likely to be much more difficult than I expected. For starters, what I never realised when I began this quest – what you can't tell from your average YouTube video – is that it's just about impossible to know how many whale sharks are out there. They can be deep-sea dwellers, with individuals tracked down further than 1900 metres. Sightings near the surface are hard to predict.

Whale sharks are even hard to find in books. In *The*

Shark: Splendid Savage of the Sea, Jacques-Yves Cousteau and his son Philippe dedicate a rare chapter to the creature, with the title, 'Peaceful Giant'. I comb through and discover this description: 'Although their shape is monstrous, the whale sharks are not likely to harm a diver with their mouth, but a stroke of their powerful tail could bear disastrous consequences.'

That doesn't sound entirely like a 'peaceful' fish to me. But thoughts of 'disastrous consequences' are not the only reason I keep returning to this chapter. The reason it sticks in my mind is the revelation, from Philippe, that his father, 'in all his long career as a navigator, has encountered this enormous animal only twice.'

When searching online for images of 'whale shark dives', it's easy to get the impression that one only has to float in certain waters to see a fully grown whale shark eventually drift past. But I'm discovering more and more accounts that suggest this is far from the case.

The latest statistics from the IUCN (the International Union for Conservation of Nature and Natural Resources) tell the story of a fish in decline. Two major subpopulations of the whale shark species exist, the report states – one of the Atlantic, and one of the Indo-Pacific – and between them the numbers are split at a ratio of roughly 1:3. Over seventy-five years, the report continues (apparently three generations in whale shark terms), datasets show a decline in the Indo-Pacific region of between 40 and 92 per cent. In the Atlantic, meanwhile, the decline has been about 30 per cent. A 2005 IUCN assessment declared the species 'vulnerable'. By 2016 the species was 'endangered'.

Not for the first time, feelings of guilt stir within me. I'm ashamed to be scared of something so vulnerable. And yet, when I picture myself alone with a whale shark, fear and revulsion take over. I try to bring my thoughts back to statistics. Concentrate on the facts.

It would seem that trying to pin down what's happening with whale sharks is not a straightforward task. At one spot in Belize, for example, mean sightings fell from about five per day in the three years before 2001, to less than two per day in 2003. In the Azores, on the other hand, sightings have actually increased since 2008, probably due to a rise in water temperature. Global warming, it would appear, is making an unpredictable fish even more so.

These reports are based primarily on sightings, so are restricted to what the human eye sees in the right place at the right time. The only global database, Wildbook for Whale Sharks, has identified over ten thousand individuals so far. There may be many more thousands out there. There may not.

On a rainy day in the shed – no, Summer Pavilion – I embark on a spot of whale shark arithmetic. I start generously, imagining that there are currently fifteen thousand whale sharks patrolling our oceans – five thousand more than Wildbook has identified so far. In human terms, fifteen thousand individuals would barely make up a town, let alone fill a decent-sized corner of the ocean. But whale sharks are bigger than humans, as we know.

This prompts me to do some spurious calculations.

Using the upper brackets of whale shark length, height and width from Wikipedia, I work out that adult whale sharks have a volume of about 40 metres cubed (except that they don't – this figure would be true only if they were cube-shaped. I'm being spurious). Taking in my own upper brackets of length, height and width, I have a (less spurious, though still spurious) volume of 0.144 metres cubed. Which is 138.89 times smaller than the volume of a whale shark.

Theoretically, these values mean that a town of fifteen thousand whale sharks could potentially take up 138.89 times more space than a town of the same number of replica Georgies. If we multiply fifteen thousand by 138.89, we get a town with the equivalent size of 2,083,350 humans in volume terms, which is less than a quarter of London's total size.

What I have discovered here is mathematical proof that if all the whale sharks in the world reached their maximum cubic volume at once, and stacked themselves into the various bars, cafés, apartments and parks of central London, the rest of the world could still go for walks in Richmond and beyond.

Or, to look at it another way, if I believe the first result on Google about the volume of the oceans being 1.332 billion cubic kilometres, and, for whatever reason, I stick to my calculation putting the volume of *every* whale shark in existence at 40 metres cubed, the whale shark population takes up 0.00000045 per cent of the volume of the world's oceans. Which is significantly more than I do, but not much. At least it doesn't look like much. Which is reassuring in terms of being a phobic who wants to avoid the big fish. But not in terms of being a phobic who's aiming to track one down.

I had thought it would be simple to come across something that big in the water. Especially given the number of businesses selling whale shark tours – more and more each time I look. After all, it's not just the whale shark's size that must be eye-catching for spotters. Their markings are flamboyant patterns of the type you could expect to see splashed over a seventies-era pleather sofa set. Jazzy, crowded, striking: these patterns might be depicting a prehistoric vision of the universe, with circular stars and the streaks of burning meteors. When I focus on pictures of them I start to suspect that, if you put all the world's whale sharks together, connecting them like pieces in the world's most ludicrous jigsaw, their markings would combine to map out the location of another dimension: the planet from which they first came, or the alien void they travel to when they leave the surface behind.

In the end, to my astonishment, it is not a poorly brewed cup of Sunshine's Special Coffee™ which terminates my stay with the ladies. Nor is it the suggestion from Sunshine that I've been casting spells to make it rain and thus avoid all work except for her memoirs. Instead it is an ivy bush that, apparently, I've trimmed wrong. It goes like this: I'm standing on top of a ladder, smartening the ivy bush as requested, when Sunshine parks herself on a garden chair and starts to shout at me. She tells me what I'm doing is not OK. That I've 'ruined everything.' I apologise, descend from the ladder and wonder what has happened. When I move the ladder Sunshine shrieks.

Luna bursts out of the house.

'I don't know what she's *doing*, Luna. Didn't you *tell* her?'

I look at Luna. She looks at me. This morning she's come out twice to see how the work on this bush has been going. Not once has my ivy technique received any criticism. The two of us could be allies in this. *Come on, Luna*, I telepathise. *Do the right thing.*

'I'm upset, Luna! I'm upset!' Sunshine shouts.

In response, Luna stammers and flusters. She anchors her hands to her hips.

'Will you two girls just get on here without me?' she says.

The statement makes Sunshine even more furious. We are getting nowhere.

'I'm sorry,' I say. 'I've stopped now. I'll clear it all away. I just thought you wanted—'

'She's so *insolent*,' shouts Sunshine. 'It's not all about *you*.'

I feel like I'm about to snap. 'I think I'd better go home,' I say.

'She's so up herself, Luna!' screams Sunshine. 'She's so up herself!'

The moment has finally come. A few hours and some changes of transport later, I stagger out at Victoria station, into the arms of Ted, and veer between laughter and wanting to punch a wall.

I'm back where I started. *Again*.

Perhaps this is what happens when one chooses land over sea. Perhaps I should build a career on leaving the land behind me altogether. Like the man who drove my coach back to London. I'm still not sure how we came on to the subject, but in no time at all the two of us were ensconced in a conversation about diving. It was as if the sea had charged us with its currents, like the driver had sensed it in me, and I in him.

He used to be a diver in the Navy, he told me. And those were the best years of his life. 'I went to the Falklands, took out some quad bikes, drove around the island. Me and the guys found a bunch of elephant seals all in a row and ran across them. They [the seals] were furious!'

He told me that, as a naval diver, he once found a formal loophole stating that he was the only person aboard who was allowed to bathe in the captain's bath – apart from the captain, of course – and that he used to redeem that privilege regularly, to the envy of his shipmates. He said that one day he was ordered down to retrieve a broken anchor from the sea floor, but when his seniors told him the depth he should reach, he worked out it would kill him. He refused and got out of the water, directly disobeying the command – and receiving no punishment for it. The coach driver told me that he would sometimes dive in oil tanks to make repairs, feeling his way through a pitch-black slick, methodically, without fear. Then, as we queued up at a roundabout, he told me about the time he was called upon to aid an American naval vessel.

'This ship had just crossed the Atlantic,' he said, 'and it arrived in Britain with one member of crew gone missing. I was asked to have a look and see if I could find him. They sent me to the freshwater tank – you know, the tank that supplies all the drinking water onboard. I got in there and did my checks and that's where I found him. Turns out one of his fellow crew members had murdered him and chucked his body in there. And he'd been there for a while. *Everyone* onboard had been drinking that water the whole time.' The driver laughed.

Intrigued and needing distractions, I take a chance while Ted is out to look up other jobs that professional divers can do; what I might be able to do once I successfully vanquish my fears. The best paid by far is saturation (or sat) diving, a job that involves spending up to twenty-eight days at a time inside a controlled, pressurised chamber of rooms within a ship or oil platform. The chamber's heavily regulated pressure levels enable everyone inside it to work in deep water for far longer than they could if they had to return to surface pressure after every dive – buying them up to eight hours of dive-time a go, in fact; enough time to patch pipelines, fix joints, etc. (Most recreational dives, by contrast, last no more than an hour.) As a sat diver pressured to a simulated depth of 100 metres, you can pop in and out of the sea at that depth without problems, no need for your body to decompress before drying off, taking a break, and preparing to go back in.

I learn that, unless Ted and I move to Aberdeen, the chances are I won't meet many divers who have this kind of relationship with the ocean. But that any I do encounter will be on a handsome salary, possibly earning more than £1000 for each day that they work.

Except that living for a month inside a pressurised chamber on a ship or offshore platform, only escaping to weld underwater, or deal with leaking pipes, has to be one of the riskiest career moves going. As soon as you are sealed into the chamber along with the rest of your team, a mixture of gases is pumped into the airtight space around you, preparing your body to properly function at depth. Helium is one of those gases, and means that divers inside the chamber quickly sound like Mickey Mouse with his testicles trapped in a vice. Meanwhile, if something goes wrong inside that chamber it could take up to five days to decompress and get the occupants out to safety.

My mother calls to check up on me. I tell her what I've been reading, and she reveals she knows a sat diver based out in Sydney, a dive-mad ex-pat called Bruce who she met in her twenties. If I want to know more about the job, she's sure he'd be happy to talk. At the very least he might have some useful tips for dealing with sea-based fears.

Another diver lurking in plain sight. Look closer and they are everywhere.

Mum sources an email address for him that afternoon and I write. Soon Bruce and I are planning a time for a video chat. But first he wants to let me know that he has been involved in sat diving for almost forty years, and retired only very recently. After giving me an overview of his experience, he writes in passing that, these days, he gets his kicks from sailing around the Pacific. He wants to check, once I've read through all this, whether having a chat is still of interest to me. After all, I mentioned wanting to know about things like sharks and fear, but, says Bruce, 'I only had a couple of nearly terminal experiences during my career.'

My interest, I tell him, is huge.

Diverted by a run of sat-diving research, I see whales

almost knock divers from their platforms, plus the pieces of a man who'd literally burst: a victim of the notorious Byford Dolphin accident of 1983, in which an exterior attendant opened a door to the diving bell (a metal chamber which carries its occupants between sea level and the depths) before the divers leaving it had been fully secured in their own compressed ship's quarters. The pressure around them plummeted in a split second, from nine bars (equivalent to 90 metres' depth) to one bar (surface level). All four divers died instantly; some explosively. The force killed the attendant too, while parts of the diver nearest the door – a Norwegian aged just thirty-four – were found ejected some 10 metres from the bell. Bruce would have been sat diving himself when that happened, as would many other divers like him. Surely these people are skilled at managing panic, in the water, in life, in all things. I'm impatient to find out how.

After several false starts, technical issues in which neither of us can hear what the other is saying, eventually Bruce and I come to a savvy arrangement of visuals through one app and audio through another. The camera slightly below him, Bruce is cast in shade, sitting in a room bathed in green light. I, meanwhile, am having issues with my chair, and am stuck in my seat peering up at the camera. A child before the guru.

I've no idea where to begin. This is a man who has been down as far as 165 metres under the water to work on the sea floor. Who has spent no less than thirty-four days in one go living at pressure – a length of time no longer considered safe by today's standards. Bruce has worked in the cold North Sea, the tropical shores off Borneo, the vast Indian Ocean, and just about everywhere else besides. I want to know everything all at once. I want to know his scariest moments: what led him there and how he overcame them.

But you cannot go straight to the hard stuff every time.

Instead we begin with the softer topics. Squeaky voices, for instance. I ask if the divers get used to them after a while. Bruce says that, yes, they do, mostly. Though a couple of his friends once worked at 265 metres, where the gas mix needed to survive made their voices so high that no one – no one – knew what they were saying; not the external support team, nor their fellow divers. 'They just gave up,' says Bruce. 'They couldn't understand each other.'

Next I ask about the food that is passed to them in the chamber. Is it true that you can't taste anything at high pressure? Bruce nods – tells me he used to add chilli sauce to every meal he had down there. It's probably why he has stomach problems now, he laughs.

I laugh too. Then decide to press on with more serious matters. If you can't taste the food, I say, can you still smell farts?

'Most definitely you can,' he says. I put a tick and write *Can smell farts*, glad to have it covered.

What about the toilet? How do the toilet things happen?

Bruce bears with me, patiently. He tells me that going to the toilet is a two-person manoeuvre, involving close coordination with external support staff.

'It's a major operation,' he explains. 'It involves you and the life-support technician [one of the external team that's on standby, 24/7, to make sure the divers have everything they need]. The toilet has an inch-and-a-half-thick lid on it, so you do your business and put this lid down – that closes the valve – and then you open another valve and flush it into a little holding tank, close that valve and open another valve, and then the guy on the outside's got two valves as well. Even taking a piddle is a bit of a drama.'

In a sat dive there's no such thing as privacy, and for some, Bruce tells me, that moment of the blowdown – when, at the start of a job, still at surface, the chamber doors lock and the atmosphere becomes pressurised – a real personality change can kick in.

'I'm not sure whether it's confinement, the heliox [a breathing gas of helium and oxygen commonly used for deep dives], the fact that you've really lost control of your life, or a combination of the three. You wouldn't know some blokes were "in the bin" for twenty-eight days,' he says, 'but some become really demanding and whingy. Constantly pushing the call button for something or other.'

Typically you will share a cramped pressurised chamber with eleven other divers for up to four weeks. The last four or five days of this will be pure decompression time. In the twenty-three days or so while you're out at depth, you and your fellow sat divers will take it in turns to work in groups from the diving bell, drilling, fixing holes, labouring, making technical corrections, whatever it is that needs doing.

But even before the bell is lowered from the ship into the water, just connecting and moving through to it is a process that could kill everyone inside, as it did the diving crew of the Byford Dolphin. Once everything's deemed to be airtight and safe, once your group is in, the bell is lowered into the water from the ship, which uses all its thrusters to stay stable at the surface. When divers pass out of the bell and into the depths, they remain attached to the bell by an 'umbilical', a lead of up to 70 metres in length that not only acts as the breadcrumbs to take them back to relative safety, but feeds them the right mix of gases, pumps hot water through their suit, monitors the pressure, and – often, but not always – provides a communication channel with their support divers. If any part of the umbilical disconnects, a diver will find themselves minutes from death at the most. Like Bruce's friend who was working in Norway when the hot water stopped flowing through his suit. In the time it took him to swim the 70 metres back to the bell, he could feel himself losing consciousness from hypothermia. (He survived.)

Bruce has had a couple of near-misses too – those 'nearly terminal experiences'. Once, when he was testing it, a gas bottle exploded, tearing through his cheek and lower teeth (he taps on his falsies, grinning). The other near-miss happened when he was working at 50 metres somewhere off the coast of Ecuador. 'My umbilical parted,' he tells me. 'I was so covered in thick grease that I couldn't undo my safety valve [to release a backup supply of emergency air] so I had to do a free ascent from 50 metres.'

Ascending from 50 metres is easily fatal for someone who doesn't have time to stop and adjust to the pressure change. It was nearly fatal for Bruce. 'I don't remember the last 20 metres,' he says. 'I lost consciousness. I was brought up by a stand-by diver and came to on the deck.'

The incident did not stop him diving, however. Almost nothing could. Bruce was a rigger in the earliest days, when sat deaths were common, the equipment was unreliable and some supervisors 'just weren't up to speed', putting their crews in unnecessary danger, occasionally giving men jobs they hadn't been properly trained to perform. Like almost all sat divers, Bruce routinely dived in zero visibility, seeing with his 'ten eyes' – a sat diving term for his fingers. He worked for up to six hours per shift in waist-high mud, under pressures so intense that his body felt close to breaking. Like many sat divers Bruce has also been in close proximity to tragedy. He tells me about one event that has always stayed with him, a catastrophe near Hong Kong that led to the death of four diver friends. Later I look up the details and find an article from the archives of the *Los Angeles Times*. It was published on 16 August 1991, and describes the capsizing and sinking of a barge carrying almost two hundred oil pipeline workers. The

barge had been struck by a typhoon, and, at the time the article was written, four sat divers were trapped, still alive but out
of reach, in a diving bell on the floor of the South China Sea.

Their air supplies were quickly running out. 'Diving
experts searched feverishly for the chamber,' states the article,
'in wild seas about 65 miles southeast of Hong Kong.'

On hearing the news that they'd gone missing, Bruce and
his team steamed across to Hong Kong to help, but were pre-
vented from joining the rescue by their insurance companies.
'That was horrible,' he says. 'Really horrible. Knowing that
four of your mates . . . ' He trails off.

Even this did not deter him from spending up to six weeks
away from home at a time, becoming a man his wife referred
to as 'the lodger'. I want to know why it didn't. How he
coped, when so many others might well succumb to fear – or
common sense.

'I think you just keep looking at your wallet,' Bruce laughs.
Then, more seriously, 'I guess I didn't think about it too
much.' He was too busy, he elaborates. Concentrating on the
work in hand.

Bruce could only hold the thoughts back for so long.
During one particularly grim placement in Borneo, when
the water was black and the mud was high, his mind began
to protest. 'I started to think about being in the chamber. And
the fact that I couldn't get out. I started to think, even if I spit
the dummy it's still going to take me five days to get out of this
bloody place. I started to really think about it. And the more I
thought about it – I think I talked myself into a stress attack.'

I ask if somebody said something that put him off. Or was
there another near-terminal event? Did more of his friends
get killed?

Bruce shakes his head. 'I just talked myself into not liking
it any more,' he says. 'It was hard luck.' That was to be his last

run of sat dives. After that Bruce moved to external duties, becoming a life-support technician, attending to the divers' every need from outside the confinement of the chamber.

Our conversation leaves me with a thought that won't go away: that the tide of the mind can turn at any moment. That no matter how experienced or confident you may be, sometimes an impulse arises that can't be quelled.

In London, where there are no big fish, no diving bells, no ivy bushes, and people (usually) say what they mean without shrieking, my living situation's more comfortable than it has been for a while. Ted and I are making efforts to have fun, hang out, be a couple. But at the same time there are new threats to our stability. Ted is going to be made redundant from his customer service job, he has learned. He's typically laid-back about it; says he feels OK. The package he'll get will support him while he finds another job. Or maybe he'll apply for a funded PhD – begin another creative writing course.

'Great idea,' I say. 'Where would you do it?' This is the crucial question, the *Get Out Of London At Last* card, but after a couple of weeks of research Ted mentions he likes the look of Goldsmith's, maybe Royal Holloway. Both are a short commute from where we live now. Neither would give us a reason to leave the city.

Having decided myself against a life on oil rigs – too messy, too dark, too perilous – I propose other places where the two of us could live together. Not Shropshire, but alternatives with other universities Ted might enjoy, within easy reach of London and his friends. Nothing I say wins him over, and, after a while, the process of even asking him elicits an instant grimace. Seeing no other way forward, and worrying I've been too bullish, I relent.

'Fine,' I say. 'Let's move in with your friends. Just as long as we find a place with a big room. And lots of privacy. Somewhere really quiet, that doesn't feel like London.'

Ted looks surprised. 'I thought you hated the house-share idea.'

'I do, but I'm willing to give it a go.'

'Hmm.' He rubs his beard. 'I'm not sure it'd work though.'

'What other choice do we have?'

He shrugs. Looks sad. 'I don't know. Let's keep thinking.'

It feels like something awful is on the horizon, but neither one of us wants to believe it. We do what most people do when they approach a frightening turning point in their lives: continue to avoid the biggest issue, diverting ourselves with what seem like more manageable goals. While Ted uses up his last weeks in the office casting the net for PhDs, I focus on how great it would be to address fear and big fish, just to tick that one off the list. We both need to feel as if we're working towards something achievable. And in the meantime, at the end of every day, the two of us take refuge in each other.

When Ted isn't there to talk to, I tell anyone who'll listen that I'm going round in circles, getting nowhere. I'm a raft emitting distress signals. One cousin, who works at an airline, hears I'm drifting. He calls to say that, if I want, he can book me an ultra-cheap flight to Florida. I could use a small piece of the savings I've tried to accumulate for a house deposit to go to a family wedding that's planned out there, then do some more diving afterwards. I'm not sure. I worry that Ted might mind me leaving again.

In fact, it doesn't seem to faze him. 'No stress,' he says. 'You do what you have to do.'

'Want to come too?'

'It's OK,' he says. 'I have applications to keep me busy.'

'Are you sure?'

He darts behind me, slots his arms under my armpits, and

scoops me up; a ticklish move guaranteed to make me laugh. 'Swiiiiim!' he cries. 'Be freeeee!'

My new plan of action lifts a weight off us both. As long as I'm not panicking about my daily routine. As long as it stops me moping. As long as it postpones my troubling questions on when and how we're going to move forward.

I book the flight and read up on the diving in Florida. Whale sharks sometimes inhabit the northern waters, I learn, but not at this time of year. Instead I can dive with bull sharks. *Yes. I could dive with bull sharks.* They may not be the biggest, they may not be what I have in mind when I think about my main purpose, but they'll surely teach me something about how I can cope with fear.

Perhaps this will be a handy sub-quest to keep me on track. It's the kind of sub-quest I'm willing to attempt. Because these sharks will test my phobia without testing how I fit into the world. Because bull sharks are uncomplicated. Because swimming with bulls is a popular niche in the market, frequently tried and tested, even by the numerous divers I've met at James Deane's shop. Because Sharkopedia says they are 'heavy sharks that aggressively take what they want, when they want it, and I envy that.'

Because I don't know what else to do.

Now I can fill my time by comparing insurance providers. Finding myself an outfit for the wedding, and further researching bull sharks. I can use my brain for absorbing new information – like how bull sharks can grow to more than 3.5 metres from nose to tail. How they break the scales at over three times the weight of the average British woman. How they are one of the most feared shark species around. And how, according to some sources, they are responsible for the largest proportion of shark-on-human attacks, more even than their great white relations.

Hmm.

During these preparations, in a chat about my lurch towards diving with bull sharks, a friend raises the subject of the death drive, a phrase I keep mis-spelling:

Death drive;

Death dive;

Death die.

'Could be worth considering,' she says knowingly. 'Have a read.'

The next morning I put down the bull sharks and focus on that. 'The goal of all life is death,' proposes Freud in *Beyond the Pleasure Principle.* '[T]he whole life of instinct serves the one end of bringing about death.'

Ego instincts lead to death, says Freud. Sex instincts lead to life. It's self-destruction versus self-preservation. I stop to ponder the idea that my shark and diving obsessions are all about ego and death. Does that mean part of me is really opposed to sex and life? I guess that, lately, Ted and I haven't been having too much sex. I wonder if that means we're speeding more quickly towards our deaths. If it means I'm a massive egoist. Either way I'd better do something about it. I remember Luna and Sunshine's tarot reading: how selfish they reported I was being; how they said that something major was going to go down in the spring.

I'd forgotten about that prediction. My nerves briefly turn piano-wire tight. But we're coming into autumn now. Spring is a little way off.

Five days before I'm due to leave for Florida, I head down alone to Poole, to spend another weekend with Mum and Granny Codd. In the past few weeks since I formed a plan around bull sharks, things have been better than ever between Ted and me. We're having more fun, sometimes nude fun, and our Friday morning goodbye is a happy one. Non-fraught.

Granny sits in her room alone, still unwilling to socialise with just about all of the residents around her. 'They're too old,' she complains to anyone daring to raise the subject again, despite the fact she must now be among the Top Five Oldest Residents in the building. We tell her there is a man playing a keyboard in the lounge. All her neighbours are down there, we say, and they're loving it. Granny pulls a face and shakes her head. I can see that her bad mood is not an act. It's been a while since she was upbeat. A while since she told any stories, or even mentioned happy animals at her window. I remember the Granny who picked me up from school every afternoon, collecting unusual leaves and seeds, talking about her day, playing games with words. She always had someone to see, or something to do, even if that was only returning the latest pair of jeans to M&S. Today, Granny Codd seems exhausted, first and foremost. She doesn't want to leave her armchair. Doesn't want to look at the sea or eat a Solero. I wonder if this is what terminal purposelessness looks like.

As we sign out of the nursing home, Mum tells me that the doctor wants to put Gran on antidepressants. I wish I could take her away from here and cheer her up myself.

During my second day on the coast, the sun is out and so is Mum. I don't want to stay at home alone in case I start thinking seriously about bull sharks, or anything else related to fear and dying. Instead I decide to revive my old bike and cycle down to see Granny again. Perhaps I can share a few chocolate digestives with her, motivate her with an Attenborough documentary. If it's one about sharks, I'll say, 'Look, Gran, one of those might kill me soon', and she can reply, 'Oh, you are silly. You'll be fine.' Afterwards I will go to the beach, paddle in the placid waters, tell myself that, *Granny's right. I'll be fine. All of us will be fine.*

As I pull the bike from the corner of Mum's study, I feel positive. So positive I am humming. I hum as I inflate the misshapen tyres, re-screwing the handlebars back together. Hum, hum, hum, as I scrape off the rust and work on making the saddle stay in position. The brake pads are snagging against my back wheel but that's no problem, surely. The wheels still turn, after all. Hum, hum, hum, hum. Almost as an afterthought, I grab an old cycling helmet, already resenting the way it'll grease up my hair, but sensing that this bike might not be quite the trusty steed it used to be.

Two minutes later I'm teetering out of Mum's road. The wheels are making strange noises but we're going all right. We're off and heading for Granny.

Five minutes after that I'm cresting the brow of the longest hill in town. I'd forgotten about this hill but it'll be fine, I'll just coast my way down, no problem.

Don't think, Georgie, just go.

Ten seconds after that I'm going fast. I tap the brakes to slow things down. There are cars on my tail. They overtake me, followed by a bus. Shit, I am going fast. And this bike can't seem to stay in a straight line.

Twenty seconds after that things have improved: we're almost at the bottom of the hill. I speed up to get past the traffic lights.

Then I hear a loud bang. The bike is down but I am no longer on it. I am in the air. My eyes are welded shut and I'm flying in space and I know, I just know, that the trajectory I'm on will not end well.

9

Left in the Cold

'When you begin to shiver continuously, get out of the water immediately, dry off and seek warmth.'

HEAT LOSS UNDERWATER,
PADI OPEN WATER MANUAL, 1999–2007

I have broken my wrist and ribs on the tarmac. I need surgery to clamp a piece of titanium to my bones. Without it my left thumb will be rendered useless. If I hadn't been wearing a helmet I would also have broken my forehead: there is a large chunk gone from the plastic that covers the weakest section of skull. Without that plastic, my brain would now be peeping out beside my right eye like a crop of flame-coloured coral.

No shark-swimming for me.

On the plus side, when Mum and I stop off at the nursing home straight after my A&E visit, the sight of my cast rouses Granny.

'What have you done?' she exclaims. 'Have some crisps. Shall I break the other one?' I want to smile but I'm still shaking with shock. I let out a sob of self-pity instead.

Passing up Mum's offer of somewhere quiet to recuperate, I insist on catching my train back to Ted, and cower my way to London cradling an arm that's still flecked with dried plaster. A dispiriting few weeks follows. Nil-by-mouths ordered by doctors for procedures that don't happen; an operation, delayed again and again; post-surgical appointments with embittered nurses. The physio team are a friendly bunch, but the things they make me do to my wrist make me think I'll be impaired for ever. The joint won't bend like it should. It hurts. It smells weird. And whenever I attempt to laugh, broken bits of my ribs jab my lungs into submission. Regularly, I slump on the sofa bed and think about the alternative me, who is currently scoping dive shops in Palm Beach. I wonder how she's doing. If she's having an excellent time out there. If she's managed to meet a bull shark and survive. Perhaps that Georgie's obtained a new lease of life by now.

I hate her.

Perhaps alternative Georgie loses her whole arm to a bull shark. That's the showreel I play in my head after crying through my third repetition of left-hand stretches, because being *this* Georgie does not seem fair at all. The bad stuff was supposed to happen to *this* one in spring.

I look at myself as I am right now. When I set out for Thailand six months ago, I was on my way to becoming a fearless explorer. And not just any fearless explorer: Cousteau's great successor, Mach 2, *sans* super-harpoon. But I can't imagine real adventurers spend as much time whimpering on a sofa bed as I have recently.

There is one thing I can be grateful for, however: the episode has brought me and Ted very close. My boyfriend, now officially jobless, is using a lot of his newfound free time to care for me. Literally. Not that he's had much choice – if he wants the woman sharing his bed to smell of soap and not stale B.O. he has to lather and rinse me every morning. But the fact is he does it tenderly, with a lovingness and patience that's delightful. He learns to wash my hair and tie it up. To put my bra on, instead of pinging it off. He cooks all my meals, taking requests for favourites. Gives me my pills. Hides the Solpadeine when I think I might be becoming a codeine addict. He even buys me a special device that props books open, allowing me to turn the pages with my single, working hand.

Mostly I am not reading, though, and Ted – alas – can't always be there when I want him. He has degrees to apply for, proposals to write amid the stillness of the library, without a distraction like me to put him off. In this time when I cannot go out, cannot immerse myself in water, can't even wet my wound in the shower without risking infection, I start thinking more than ever about being submerged. Submerged on wrecks, in particular.

For many tec divers – James Deane, for one – it's the wrecks that make their dangerous hobby worthwhile: an exploration of once-human domains; the promise of treasure, guarded only by fish. For that they risk entanglement, air hoses snagged on shards of metal, massively diminished visibility. That small hole in the hull that led you in: can you find it now the silt is flying about you? And if your torch breaks . . . If narcosis hits . . .

There's also the question of what you might find down there. A pair of legs sticking out from the superstructure, perhaps. That's what one of James's customers saw. When he gently pulled on the corpse, a startled treasure-seeker twisted around to discover who was yanking on his leg.

My search results know how sombre I've been feeling. From the safety and dullness of land, eventually able to sit up with my laptop, I've flooded myself with stories of wreck

dives gone wrong – at the site of HMHS *Britannic*, for example, the *Titanic's* sister ship. In 1916, *Britannic* sank in the
Aegean, scuppered by a mine. It was the largest vessel lost
in the First World War. Thirty died as it went down, killed
while in two lifeboats by giant, still-whirring propellers
('churning and mincing up everything near them', as one
eye-witness put it). Naturally it was Jacques Cousteau's team
who first dived the wreck some sixty years after that. For the
intrepid crew of Cousteau's ship, the *Calypso*, the dive was a
daunting challenge. The first time they descended to the level
at which *Britannic* lay – between 40 and 80 metres from the
surface – their light bulbs exploded underwater. One of the
crew was forced to ascend, affected by narcosis. In the end, all
emerged intact, paving the way for future waves of tec divers.

Thirty-three years later, in 2009, the wreck claimed the
life of Carl Spencer, a deep-diving expert leading a project
to film there at the site. It was not his first visit to *Britannic*,
but nonetheless something went wrong with his rebreather,
a piece of deep-diving equipment that recycles the breath,
removing carbon dioxide and refreshing it with oxygen.
Carl signalled an emergency and rocketed up to the surface
from depth. He was killed by a severe case of the bends. One
account I read says he ought to have decompressed for two
hours before surfacing. Instead he had only seconds.

Continuing along this morbid path, I read about someone
who did not decompress during a deep dive in the Red Sea.
This person shot to the surface from around 130 metres, and
a physician at the local hyperbaric chamber commented that,
by the time he broke into the daylight, he 'must have been
bubbling like a Pepsi-Cola.' The image is almost ridiculous.
For a moment I can't believe it. Then I remember a story
James Deane told me about Bob, his old business partner, the
one who eventually disappeared in French waters. One day

Bob arrived at the shop and told James that his stomach felt odd. He asked if his friend would investigate.

On inspection, James heard a sound coming from under Bob's skin – a popping, 'like Rice Krispies'. Bob was bent. I have never popped like Rice Krispies. And am not likely to for as long as I sit on this sofa bed. Because while I'm on this sofa bed, 30 miles away from the nearest coast, I know that I am safe.

The thing is, as dependable as it might be, there's a problem with feeling safe. And that's that you can get stuck there very quickly. When you wake up and know how your day will pan out. That it will be just like the day before, and the day before that. When you see no alteration in your routine. I know I need stability. But I'm also starting to notice that comfort blankets can be smothering.

It turns out the situation is also troubling for Ted. After weeks of slow recovery, when I need him in the shower less and less, something in him seems to change, and not for the better. He's more and more uncertain about the idea of a PhD. He does not know what he wants to do with his time. We put the talk off for as long as we can, but once all the other major topics have been exhausted, we have no choice but to come back to the subject of where we are going to move next. The old split remains: I really want to leave the city, he would like to stay.

On Christmas Day, the two of us visit Ted's family – it's my turn since Ted came to mine last year. At several points his mother asks, in varying ways, what exactly we're going to do with ourselves next. Neither of us have an answer that makes sense. Afterwards, I propose the idea of moving abroad and trying something new together, just for a year, just the two of us.

'Sounds great,' Ted says. 'You should totally do it.'

'You', he says, not 'we'.

'I meant we'd do it together,' I clarify.

'That's not my thing, Gogs,' says Ted.

A couple of days after that we travel to Dorset. Neither Granny nor Mum asks about our plans – Granny's distracted by back pain; Mum's engrossed in a new job – and we're relieved not to have to go through the same discussions again. Instead we can focus on things that might pep Granny up, like bringing her baked bean fritters from the chippy, or showing her endless pictures of dogs and Prince George. For Ted and I an impasse has never seemed less unavoidable, but talking it through just makes us both feel worse. And soon, worse is how things get.

January comes, and with no promising leads to tempt him one way or another, nothing to reward all the emails and ideas he's been working on, Ted becomes upset, frustrated, hopeless. Watching his ego corrode, I decide I'll nurse us back to health by pepping him up too, repaying his kindness from when I was most broken. I start by making his favourite meals. I offer massages. Buy all the best baked goods I can find. Wear my fanciest knickers. At the same time, I stop posing any more questions about our future, giving him the peace he seems to crave. But, despite my best efforts, it soon becomes clear that I don't have the power to heal this. I am too much a part of the problem.

When I'm alone in our flat, when Ted returns to his parents, in search of more room to think, I fantasise about being back in the waters of Thailand; that this whole situation is a shipwreck to explore. Sadness is not a part of me then. I'm just a floating observer.

I think of the life clustered around the wreck of the *Boonsung*, an ex-mining vessel we stopped at on our way home from Richelieu Rock. I saw rock-like devil scorpionfish there, walking across the sand like missing links. Through a gap in the ship's metal frame I watched a school of squid hovering over us. Distant. Harmless. Bizarre. Later, a fist-sized pufferfish deflated before our eyes, shrinking a little with each reverse jerk through the water. Its spikes reverted to smoothness. Its bright eyes went wide again.

Sometimes destruction can lead to amazing things.

Then I think of the wreck of the *Premchai*, the final dive I had. I remember how the blue visibility vanished; how all of us were swept up in a whirl of underwater sand, unable to see more than a couple of metres in front of our faces. I remember how we scrabbled around the hull, shielding ourselves from the power of the tide.

Destruction leading to chaos.

Full disintegration, without distractions, breaks Ted and me apart in a matter of weeks. At the end, I still think we could make things work. Ted disagrees. More than six years as a couple gone. I can't face it. Even as he is saying his final I Love You and last Goodbye, I spy a barren hinterland of an after-math and veer myself away. *Lah lah lah, this isn't happening.*

It's winter. It's bleak. It seems obvious that keeping moving is essential. I'm sure that if I falter without purpose I'll break down myself, so I stir up as much as I can to keep myself occupied. I need to find a new place to live. Maybe find myself a mate. Not to mention a whale shark. I must achieve a whale shark. Deal with the king of the fish. But first I need to get my income sorted. Fast.

With no better options available at short notice, I reluc-tantly ask for a permanent job at the clinic I worked in before I left for Thailand. My former employers say yes. It feels like a wrenching step backwards, but will have to do for the moment. Meanwhile, during my daily updates to Mum,

I hear that Granny Codd is not doing well. She has been sleeping almost all the time for the past few days, my mother reports. 'She has a bad infection. When that goes she should get better. You know Granny. She always bounces back . . .' I want to come down to see her. I ask if I should come down right now.

'I'm not sure you need to,' says Mum. 'I'll keep you posted. There's not that much you can do.'

I can't lose Granny too. That isn't allowed.

What I wish I could do instead of bracing myself for more bad news is head out again and dive; continue to prove I can dilute my fears, even if they're only the fears that relate to fish and other sea creatures. But I know I can't fly away from home this time. Instead I'd better at least attempt to rebuild my life in England first, and keep myself a train ride away from Granny.

When I do visit her she is wilting, just like Mum implied. She's not keen to talk much. Not able to stay out of bed for too long.

'I want to go home,' she whispers to me, her watery eyes fixed on mine. '*Please*. Would you just take me home?'

'I can't,' I say. 'You need people to look after you.'

Granny Codd scowls. She insists that she doesn't.

'You might hurt yourself,' I tell her, but the argument seems feeble. Granny is already hurting. Why shouldn't she hurt in the place she used to live; in the home she actually likes? I should offer to look after her – she's looked after me enough times. Years of looking after me, in fact. I feel the urge to say I'll quit the clinic and move to Dorset. But I'm too scared. Granny is no longer full of tales and treats. She is somebody old and falling apart, who needs to be bathed and changed. She's a fragile, full-grown adult. *I* could end up hurting her. I could end up *hating* her. I change the conversation, trying to keep her mind off the situation. Granny plays along for a while and then closes her eyes. I start to leave as she's drifting off.

'I have to catch my train now,' I say softly.

Immediately she comes to. 'When are you coming back next?' she asks.

'As soon as I can.'

'Oh.'

I rack my brains for something that might validate my departure. 'I'm working on a project in London,' I say.

'Yes?' She widens her eyes. 'Are you?'

'It's about fear and scuba diving. It's keeping me pretty busy.'

'Oh,' says Granny. She smiles. 'That's nice.'

Coward, Georgie. You are such a coward. Although it is true that my project is keeping me busy. That's how I am structuring it. That's what I want it to do.

It is during this frenzied period that I am most drawn to James Deane's shop, where I can have adventures by proxy. James's stories of death and diving scratch an itch I can't reach anywhere else at the moment. His world is a world with real danger. Raw fight-or-flight responses. Where love lives and urology clinics and home nursing don't feature. Where social obligations have little importance. Where all are small fish encircled by bigger ones. And where, even in situations of major trauma, it's still possible to stay calm. As long as you know, or think you know, what you're doing.

'You have to meet Mungo,' James tells me. 'Mungo's got some great stories.' But he doesn't think I should meet Mungo just because of his great stories. He wants me to meet Mungo because Mungo often dives without a buddy, totally on his own in caves and quarries, down to depths that would quickly put an end to a novice like me. Talking to Mungo would help me understand fear all the better, James believes.

So many of the deaths I've heard of so far have involved divers swimming alone, whether diving solo on purpose, or cleaved from their group by unexpected circumstances. Like Yuri Lipski, the man who filmed his own demise at the Blue Hole. Like Dave Shaw, a record-breaking Australian diver who got caught up in the kit of a dead body he was retrieving. Like Peter Verhusel, who lost his buddies, lost his way and starved to death after three weeks alone on a pitch-black cavern ledge.

When I picture myself encountering the whale shark, I always picture meeting it on my own, irretrievably separated from whoever brought me there, hanging in miles of blank water like a slow-motion marionette. Me, the shark and oblivion. A moment that cuts the strings that hold me in place. Is Mungo not scared to go solo?

'I have a healthy fear for everything I do,' he says, when we meet at a pub in Peckham. Recently that included diving solo to a depth of 106 metres at a flooded slate quarry in Wales – a quarry with the deceptively friendly name of Dorothea. The water there, he tells me, was two, three degrees. No one else was in it. All that waited for him in the deep was a sign attached to a wall depicting a smiley face, along with a greeting, 'WELCOME TO THE BOTTOM OF DOTTY', and instructions on how to return to the surface. Mungo filmed the whole dive from his helmet. Silt flies not long after he reaches the floor, stirred up by the motion of his fins. Visibility ebbs.

Between 1994 and 2016, twenty-five people died at Dorothea. Most of them were divers – along with a handful of swimmers and walkers who accidentally fell in – all engulfed by the same site that Mungo flowed through on his own, completely unharmed. More than two-and-a-half hours after he entered the water, he surfaced there in one piece, not lost, not bent, not hypothermic, not drowned.

'The time flew by,' he says. 'I felt a sense of connection with the place.' And despite the quarry's history of tec diving fatalities, the only nervousness he felt down there was when something unseen touched his shoulder. He now thinks it was probably the shot-line, a rope that stretches from surface to floor, allowing a diver to find their way back to safety. But for a moment, when it happened, he wasn't sure what it might be.

Mungo seems like a sociable man. He teaches diving and motorcycling and has thousands, genuinely thousands, of Facebook friends. Beneath his massive ginger beard – 'I needed a pet, something I can take with me when I travel' – his expression conveys either merriment or wonder. When one of the pub's regulars, a tipsy bloke called Dennis, asks to join us ('Can I show her?' he asks Mungo, before poking the solid iris of his own glass eyeball), the conversation slides amusingly into an orgiastic chat about drinking, diving and, well, orgies. (Dennis: 'I've seen a man who pinched his nipples for so long he lactated. The jet of milk shot right across the room.')

With that many friends around him, I want to know why he continues to take the risks of going solo; to repeatedly head for places of danger with nobody by his side.

'Recently it's been that no one else wants to do what I want to do,' Mungo says. 'Too deep, too cold, too weird.'

Besides, he adds, some sites insist that you dive them without any buddies. That way you're only responsible for yourself. Your air, your lines, your escape. No one's there to block your way out, or hamper the progress you're making. When he's under the water, alone, Mungo feels like he's pulling off a heist. Charmed. Exhilarated. But he says the best divers aren't in it for ego or kicks. They're humble. 'They know the point of stress – and when to back out.'

There are, Mungo says, 'great moments of connection when things go well. Like in exploration cave dives where you almost close your eyes because you're that mellow with it. Not through nonchalance but because it's calming. It's intoxicating.'

Though these beatific connections don't always happen. Mungo tells me about one cave dive during which he could not find his markers or line back up to safety. Another group of divers had mistakenly packed them away. 'I went past the point of no return for gas,' he tells me. 'For about fifteen minutes I thought, *I'm going to die.*'

I want to know how that felt. What it's like to have to confront your own death, knowing it's due in just a few gauge readings' time. Holding my half of Guinness tightly, I pose the question to him.

'Like an overwhelming mix of intense stupidity, loneliness, frustration – and a hell of an adrenaline hit,' replies Mungo. But despite those feelings he did his best to collect himself. And, in one last bid to stay alive, he made an educated guess about the way out. 'It turned out I was on the right route and the route was cool. When I saw the natural light in the cavern section – I can't describe that feeling.'

Another high-risk escapade saw Mungo trapped on a wreck alone in Egypt. 'I lost my visibility and my main post [the section between his air tanks] snagged on one of the lines. So I was stuck. And it was one of those dives where I was inside the wreck and deep, and the air consumption's massive and in this chamber, not that long before I went, a guy had died. I could exactly see why he died. It was the same thing that happened to me.'

In both of these near-misses, Mungo was able to keep his

cool while facing death and not let the fear cloud his judgment. I want to know his secret. I need to know.

'Practice, practice, practice,' he tells me. If I'm serious about
learning to dive safely, about feeling properly confident to
dive among all fish and whale sharks, I must overlearn what
I am doing. As if I'm in the military. Like the coach driver.
'Soldiers are not amazingly courageous,' Mungo explains.
'Some of them are. But most of them are very, *very* well
trained on over-learned behaviour.'

The truth is, when things go wrong, he says, divers ought
to be able to fix their problems by themselves. 'You can't rely
on your buddies,' adds Mungo.

Winter's getting bleaker. Granny Codd is significantly out
of sorts. Next time I see her she tries to talk and falls asleep
mid-sentence. The doctor has diagnosed another infection,
Mum explains. They say she'll be better after a new course
of antibiotics. It's good news, but I want her to feel better
now. I want to feel better myself. To take back some control.

Practice, practice, practice, I hear Mungo saying. On my return
journey to London, I resolve to find something short and
constructive to focus on; something that does not require a
huge commitment, or long distance. Something that might
help me with the big fish.

Arriving home, alone, to the flat that Ted will take back
when I am gone – he and his parents are letting me play
cuckoo for a few more weeks while I gather myself – I briefly
set aside the joyless hunt for a new place to live, and make
an impromptu booking for a drysuit training course: a day
that will teach me how to dive in a suit that keeps its users
warm in cold (sometimes ice-cold) water. With even the UK's
mellowest seas maintaining the low average temperatures that
they do, drysuit diving would be the best way to hone my

scuba skills over the coming months; to make myself a *sensei* of the sea, ready for whale sharks and anything else the ocean decides to throw at me.

The training takes place on a freezing Saturday in late February. It is five months since I Supermanned the pavement with my wrist, and today will be my first set of dives since the accident. My surgeon has said it's OK to go ahead. The physio team has agreed. I hope they're right. If my wrist gives out in the lake I could be in trouble. At least there won't be any predatory fish in there to contend with.

The shore swarms with a mass of trainees and instructors. Everyone's getting ready, suiting up. Except me. For fifty minutes I sit on a bench in a northerly wind waiting for my instructor exactly where I've been told to wait. It is not unlike my arrival on Koh Tao pier. Only much, much colder.

Already chilled to my core I wander around, attempting to find out where this instructor might be. A woman in a drysuit overhears me.

'Oh, you're supposed to be with us,' she says casually.

Turns out she's my instructor for today. I wish I'd known this forty-five minutes ago. I wish she had told me before I lost most of my body heat. I follow her to a van in the car park where my basket of kit is waiting, along with three other divers doing the course. Keeping my own clothes on underneath, I start to suit myself up. Then I break off and dash for the toilet. My bladder is very nervous. It knows that it can't let itself go in the drysuit. If I pee in this thing I'll be peeing on all my own clothes. And on a pricey piece of kit that I have rented from the dive school. Not, I think, a great way to make new friends. Though by this point I'm not sure that I want to make friends any more. It's too cold. I just want to get in and do the two dives I need to officially qualify. I plan to do them perfectly. With focus. With control. I have been careful with my homework preparation. I have read the pack I was told to read, several times. I am overlearning. I know that the suit itself is my buoyancy control, and that I need to keep it level and steady. I know that if my balance isn't right, the air could collect in my feet and pull me back to the surface by the ankles. I know that this could be dangerous.

I feel afraid. Afraid of doing this wrong. PADI instructions say that I shouldn't go in if I don't feel up to it mentally. Only there's lots of things I don't really feel up to right now. Like leaving the bed. Like leaving the flat. Like going back down to the nursing home. Does that mean I'm supposed to stay put at all times?

I take some breaths and distract myself by watching the people around me. The atmosphere they're projecting is a positive one. Plenty of chat, plenty of movement. No one here is crying. If anyone else is afraid right now they're keeping it well contained. Maybe because they're blokes. Not all of them, but the vast majority. They queue at the lake, city types, lads, hardened middle-aged men – not one of them my idea of a suitable new buddy – and wait their turn to dive in a banterous mood. Or maybe these blokes are not well contained at all. I'm not a bloke and it probably looks like I'm keeping my fear well contained. Maybe all of us are bordering on the hysterical right now. Maybe if one of us goes the whole lot will.

My dive group makes its approach and I follow along. With me are a portly man and his wife, as well as an actress training for roles that require diving expertise. The lake seethes and roils with air, signs of the people who entered before us. As per our instructions, I trudge down the ramp to my doom. The water today is five degrees. That's only a few degrees warmer than the seas around Antarctica. Soon we four students are floating in the shallows. I feel the bite of the temperature through my drysuit. But it doesn't feel too bad in here. Not yet.

'Right,' says our instructor from the privileged position of the ramp. 'Let's practise our surface buoyancy first.' She tells us to release some air and let ourselves sink under. I am wearing a hood to keep my head warm but it's about as effective an insulator as a plastic carrier bag. As soon as I'm under the surface the chilled water not only chews my bare face, but clamps its icy claws around my neck. It scrapes the skin of my ears and scalp, as if no hood ever existed. I bob and wince and freeze, as capable of checking my own buoyancy as an iceberg would be. My mask isn't clear either, which means the right side of my vision is blurred. And, much like the hood, which obscures the rest of my view, the gloves I've been given are so large they're letting in water.

I'm not the only one having trouble. The portly man in our group can't get under at all. He needs more weights. We all rise back to the surface and wait for supplies to arrive. And wait some more.

It takes more than thirty minutes for this issue to be sorted. Thirty minutes of treading cold water with flooded gloves and a cold head. I'm shivering like a broken fridge and we haven't even started the dive. When at last we're given the go-ahead to properly descend, the feeling is absolute torture; stabbingly cold. The water is cloudy, awash with a brown sediment that's been kicked up by the numerous other trainees who crawl through the lake. My hands are so icy and weak that I can't get the stiff air button on my chest to make me buoyant. I sink and flop at the bottom and crawl too. This is supposed to be an orientation dive, but mostly I feel disorientated. Weird squeaks and squeezes, flatulent burps of rubber, fill my ears. We are down for all of eight minutes.

When we surface and scramble back to the ramp, I am too

cold to take off my fins. The dive shop assistant – helpful, though clearly a lunatic (he is wearing shorts and flip-flops in two-degree weather) – has to pull my fins off for me. Inside my socks my feet are toeless lumps. Silently I curse my lot. This is not the orderly, optimistic day out I signed up for. I waddle to the van with as much speed as I can manage, clumsily prise off my suit with shaking fingers, and throw on every backup item of clothing in my bag. That's three pairs of socks, two pairs of trousers, three thermal vests, a padded gilet, a tracksuit top, gloves, hat, coat and an ultra-long scarf. Even then it's not enough. I retreat to the lake hut where a solitary wall heater sighs warm air at a constantly opening door.

The place is packed with other divers. A hot coffee in a polystyrene cup does nothing for me. I stand alone and shiver but am by no means the worst case here. At one table a young guy's teeth are clattering as he tightens a towel round his shoulders. Another man is deep in discussion with his teacher. He doesn't want to go down again, he says. He's going to get back on the train and go home.

I could do that. I could get back on the train. I could end this right now. Except that if I scrap the second dive, go home and do what I want to do – i.e. become the human embodiment of a duvet – I know I'll never try drysuit diving again. And then I'll have another thing to fret about. My purpose here is mastering fears, not gaining any more.

You've got to train yourself. Put it in a box.

A box. Not a duvet.

'I will not go home,' I say to the heater. 'I am going to do the second dive.' The heater continues to sigh.

If this was a story of morals and learning, of determination reaping great rewards, the resolution I've just made would make this second dive a revelation. I would find that my mighty human mind was able to control my perception of the cold. I would learn that, by overriding my gut-strong aversion to this awful lake, I could take the sting out of a scary situation. Not only that: transform that scary situation into an enjoyable, life-affirming event.

But this is not what happens. Suffused with dread, only too recently free of the shivers, I follow my group back into the water, and swim with them to a point above a submerged platform. We don't faff about on the surface this time. The instructor must sense there would be a group revolt. Instead we go straight down, performing the tasks we need to per-form to pass, such as disconnecting and reconnecting the hose that supplies our suit, a job my fingers – rendered useless by the cold – can hardly manage. Though I see the instructor's mime of applause through the murk, I have a horrible feeling the hose is still disconnected. Now I can barely stay buoyant, but somehow, on command, I manage to do the forward roll we've been told will keep our drysuits level and balanced. The instructor applauds again. Afterwards my balance is more out of whack than before. I shift and flounder. Another instructor from a different group pushes me out of his way.

On the plus side, I'm much warmer than I was during our first go. On the minus side, my breathing is now an acutely unpleasant combination of sharp and heavy. This dive feels like hard physical work, in the same way that wetsuit diving never has. When our tasks are over, the instructor signals that it's time to move on and see the 'sights' of the lake – a rusty bus, for example; a small, sunken boat. But I'm not going anywhere. I am caught on a rope. After a few frantic twists and shrugs I free myself in time to see the others speed away into the sediment. I'm lagging and they're not stopping. I try to catch up and it feels like I'm swimming through quicksand. My body is heavy and goes almost nowhere. Nothing I can press or adjust seems to make me float any easier. I briefly spy the corner of a vehicle. A drowned bus. But my progress past the drowned bus is nightmarish. It starts to feel like someone is grabbing and tugging my feet. I turn around. There's no one there. And now I seem to be rising.

Breathing fast, I try letting out air, lifting my arm to release the bubbles, just like I've been taught, like I have read. The action has no effect. Finally I realise what's happening. In all my thrashing the air has shifted down into my feet. My ankles are stuck in a pocket of gas. I'm being pulled upwards. I can't get the momentum to roll over. I thrash and panic. It's hopeless. All I can do is give in. I pop out of the water feet first, so fast it's as if the lake is squeezing me out as waste. I'm a human floater. At least I was only dragged from 4 metres, or else I might be a human floater with the bends. For a minute I struggle to right myself. By the time I manage to flip onto my back I'm exhausted. I lie in the water panting, wondering whether my group has noticed I'm gone.

I knew that this would happen. As soon as I read about how air can be siphoned into the feet of a drysuit, dragging the wearer helplessly backwards and out of the water, I knew it would happen to me.

Minutes later, I'm still floating unaccompanied, too tired to move or get annoyed that my instructor left me behind. There is plenty of time to get annoyed about that on my train ride home. In fact I will remain annoyed about it until a point many months afterwards, when I discover that her dive school has gone into liquidation, liquidation being the perfect word for a diving outfit that never had any structure. *Ha*, I will think at that point. *That's exactly what you deserve for leaving me behind to get tangled in rope. You have been justly liquefied.*

For now, I see the bubbles rising near me and feel relief. I wave and try to look calm, laissez-faire, like I meant to come out of this water feet first all along. The group must have been worried about my sudden disappearance and I don't want to add to their stress. Except it turns out I've got the wrong idea. The group wasn't worried about me at all.

'Oh,' says the instructor when I tell her what happened. 'I thought you'd just gone up with someone else.'

Who? I think. *Who else would I have gone up with?*

When we reassemble, I discover the portly man had issues too. He also couldn't keep up. He also found it a struggle. And now his tank is entirely empty of air. Somehow he has sucked down 2 litres' worth in a sixteen-minute dive at a depth of 5 metres. To empty a tank entirely is a rarity, and almost unheard of in training. It looks so bad for the dive school that the assistant, still in his flip-flops, mutters how he can't write a zero on their records. The zero is a no-no. So he fudges it. Calls it a fifty.

I cannot get out of there fast enough. That evening, during my very best duvet impression, on top of the bed Ted and I used to share, the bed he will soon reclaim, I catch sight of my legs and see that they're covered with nicks and bruises. My hands are raw: dry and blistered. But there's no one I can show them to. No one to give me their sympathy, or tell me not to go drysuit diving again.

You can't rely on your buddies, said Mungo. But a reliable buddy is exactly what I want. My own company isn't enough at the moment. There is too much headspace, too much time to frighten myself with what is just out of sight. I sign up to a handful of dating websites, aiming for a minimum number of three meetings per week. Within minutes, I connect with a musician who lives in Kent, and we arrange to have drinks in a few days' time. On the first date he tells me he's smit-ten. We kiss at St Pancras Station and my chest feels like it's going to explode. For the second date I travel to Kent, where we walk through a forest, cosy up in the nook of a pub, and share an Indian meal which he gallantly pays for. That night he artfully tricks me into meeting his parents at home. 'We'll sneak in the back,' he promises, before leading me directly through the front door, where his mother seems primed to show me countless photographs of her grandchildren. On the third date he and I meet back in London, and watch a terrible film that ends with an incoming tsunami. Before we part ways for the evening, he suggests I move south, where I can live with him, his brother and his parents. We don't reach Date Number Four.

I next start talking with a young Oxbridge professor. Gamely, perhaps insanely, he invites me to his college for our first date, and I sit among his colleagues for a three-course meal with wine. The dons either side of me seem to think I'm a fellow academic. My date doesn't correct them.

'And how do you know the professor?' they ask, before we reach the port and tins of snuff.

'I'm studying scuba diving,' I announce, grasping the first non-scandalous thought that arises. 'Did you know the professor was Open Water qualified?' Turns out the professor also has an expensive car. On his phone is a picture of a woman draped over its bonnet. I'm not sure this is the buddy for me either.

While the random assortment of dates continues, I finally tear myself out of the flat, and move in with an old school friend who lives out in the suburbs. She says I can stay on her sofa for a month. I bounce between there and the clinic, earning money, though nowhere near enough for independence. A few weeks later, a second friend offers to set me up with a bank transfer: a loan I can use to rent somewhere else and plan what I'm going to do next. Their relay of kindness gets me into spring, and before I know it, Ted and I have been apart for three whole months. Occasionally friends and family comment on how upbeat I seem. I've barely paused to consider it. I can't pause.

Until it's my mum's birthday. She and I walk in the hills overlooking the sea, taking large draughts of fresh air before we head back for an afternoon visit with Granny. On our return to the car, Mum's phone starts ringing. It's the nursing home. They tell us to come and see Granny Codd. They tell us to be quick. We race through the countryside, driving as fast as we can on the main road to town, speeding along the scythe-like curve of the harbour.

When we reach Granny she is still alive, but looks like a person in her final hours. Her skin is dull. Her breathing is laboured. She can't talk or open her eyes. The noises coming from her mouth are the noises of discomfort like liquid on the lungs. It is as if as if she is drowning in a private sea. But somehow, we notice from slight groans and nods, she can still hear what we're saying.

We try to make her comfortable. And we talk. We describe some of our favourite days. We want her to remember the beach and the ice creams. The walks. The silly jokes. All the cream teas. The spiders. The Lottery tickets. Sometimes she moans. Sometimes she flinches. Occasionally the moans sound like words, but we cannot work out what they mean. This woman was in the room when I was born. She helped my mother through labour and held her hand. She held my hand too, before I even knew what a hand was. Now I'm holding her hand and stroking her soft, heavy fingers. As I speak to her, I sense something monstrous approaching.

My eldest cousin arrives and sits with the three of us. An anxious member of staff asks if someone can run out to pick up the oral morphine Granny will need to get her through the night without more pain. They are short-staffed. I look at my cousin and Mum. No one wants to leave, but I'm the fastest runner. I volunteer.

The largest, most formidable whale sharks are always the old females, I heard recently.

Granny Codd takes her last breath when I'm out of the room.

Part Two

We Drift

Searching the drawer for some mislaid thing,
I came across, for the hundredth time,
The fat, battered writing case,
And I thought — surely I can look through it now?

Surely, after twenty years, I can look through it
Without too many sights, too much pain?

Memories tapped me on the shoulder and I
        looked around,
Looked around and stayed, looking.

That girl, sitting there, she could be my daughter.
Sitting on the end of the couch, her damp hair
        pinned in curls,
A pretty dress still over her arm.
She sits awkwardly, staring at the paper in her hand.
"Dear Madam,
    We regret to inform you that your husband
    Sergeant D. G. M— has died . . . "

She was still sitting there when dawn came
Not feeling the pain in her legs.
Just staring at the paper lying on the seat beside her.
No-one had spoken.
No-one interfered.

They just left her alone in what they called
        her grief.
But I knew she wasn't grieving.
Not yet.
She was trying so hard to grieve, trying to feel
        something. Trying to make her heart and
        mind believe
What the words had to say.

He was dead, he was already buried somewhere,
His brown, beautiful body already rotting in a heap
        of hot sand.
He was not coming back ever.
He was dead, dead.
Dead.

The days and weeks passed with
Mute solace from all around her.
But, very soon the concern gave way to
        practical thoughts:

At least she has no children to look after,
She is strong and healthy.
And she is not the only one —.

She heard not a word
But she would not, could not, be alone.

Having failed to convince herself of her loss at the
        beginning,
Now, she did not want to think about it again.

So she surrounded herself with people, strangers

Who did not sympathise.
Did not even give her a second thought.
The more hours of each day that she spent with people
The less time she had to be alone,
And the less chance there was of the truth catching
    her unawares.

She became known as The Merry Widow.
But not a soul knew how she felt or why she
        was so gay.
One day, with a party of girls and arrogant
        young airmen
She went to Dancing Ledge, where the sea laps
The rocky shelves.

Only this day the sea was tall, and rough,
        and angry.
It crashed against the rocks with a hate that
        frightened the girl.
Were these drops of water on her face the drops
That has rolled off *his* face as he had floated, dying?

The young men laughed.
They held her against the rock
Until it seemed the sea would engulf them all —
This was childish fun compared with what *they* had
        been through —
And let her go in time for them to jump clear.

That night, hours after all in the house slept
She had a dream.
She was chained by her outstretched hands to a
        dark cliff.

The wind howled and she was wet with spray.
The black seas were boiling nearer and nearer,
Higher and higher.
Her struggles freed one arm
And she was desperately trying to free the other
While the waves were now breaking over her.

She woke up to find herself
Sitting on the bed
Slashing
With frenzy
At her wrist
With a blade.
And there was blood everywhere.

Voices from the present release me from the past.
As I close the draw on the writing-case
Still unopened,
I run my finger down the long thin scars
        on my wrist.

MARGARET (GRANNY) CODD
1917–2016

10

Only One Way Out

'Any time you can't swim directly up to the surface, you're in a special situation . . . Avoid this risk entirely . . . '

OVERHEAD ENVIRONMENTS,
PADI OPEN WATER MANUAL, 1999–2007

If you're ever underwater, lost inside a wrecked ship, you know that ship was built to have an exit.

If you're ever underwater, lost inside the ocean, you know that all you need to do is head up.

Other environments are harder to escape.

My grief is a wave that won't turn flat. The peak hisses and tears, unsettling parts of me I can't see. Unless I paddle faster.

I paddle faster.

It has been seven months since Granny died, ten months since my split from Ted, and since then I've thrown myself into more trips, more dates, more interviews than ever. Depression seems to get me nowhere. Worse – it sends me backwards. I have spoken to Ted since he left. Heard about his new girlfriends. Started to grow a protective shell for each time we interact. But Granny Codd is gone for ever, and that hurt isn't healing.

I'm weighed down by the things I never said. The questions I should have asked. The changes that might have made her life worth living. It's all too much to contemplate. Distractions and continuity, on the other hand, might help me through. Distractions, continuity, and, perhaps, a man named Max. Although, right now, Max is nowhere to be seen. And that's my fault.

Days before my thirtieth birthday, I'm in a plane from Mexico City, heading for the east coast near Cancún. In July and August every year, a mass of feeding whale sharks brings the tourists pouring into this part of the world. But it's winter again. I'm way too early for that.

In the wake of Granny Codd's death, my adventure has taken a new turn, though occasionally, at a distance, I think I can still see my biggest adversary waiting. I wonder if we're moving in circles, this whale shark and I. I wonder what will happen when one of us catches up with the other.

A few months ago, I met another cave diver like Mungo: a man at James Deane's called Vas. Vas was built like Action Man, was a member of the UKMC – the UK Mine/Cave Diving Club – and told me he spent most of his weekends floating through flooded coal mines. Sheltering in James's shop, wanting to latch on to something I could truly understand, I asked Vas if he could explain the appeal of cave diving to me; if he could tell me what good might come from being trapped in a pitch-dark place.

'It's tranquil,' he answered. 'Calm.' It was also, he said, a welcome challenge for someone who craves control.

I wish I had more control.

Vas went on to describe the experience of diving caves in

Mexico. How there was something otherworldly about it. Not classically attractive, but eerie, like a moonscape.

'It's so clear,' he told me, 'your brain forgets it's swimming.'

Vas didn't dwell on the dangers. Instead he said that diving in crystal clear caves was the next best thing to flying.

Flying and forgetting.

I could see the appeal.

On the plane from Mexico City, I reread my PADI manual. It stresses that overhead environments like caves are an '*extremely hazardous* situation'. It tells me I need lots of training and special equipment. It is trying to put me off. But I have already convinced myself that this birthday I'm about to have needs to be different. I'll be thirty. Officially adult. I need to find a way to face what scares me, one fragment at a time.

Even so, '*extremely hazardous*' is a strong term.

Travelling solo leaves lots of room to think. A dangerous amount. Since I set off for the airport, I've mostly fixated on why I chose to do this on my own. Just a fortnight after Granny's death, I became serious with someone I found online. This is the man named Max. Max likes to swim and travel. Max is scared of heights. Max is also scared of diving, and of being eaten alive by what's in the water. But when I asked Max if he'd ever swim with a shark he said he would try it.

In the last few months, Max's presence has taken my mind off my grimmest memories. My grandmother, transformed into something other, almost fish-like. The blackness of a mouth that wouldn't close. Her glassy eyes drying in air. His presence has also calmed me down when I've been nervous. If I feel like my limbs are stuck to the bed he will pat my back and exclaim things like, 'You can do it!' Or sometimes, gameshow-style, he'll announce to me: 'Georgie, you're a winner!' The man is my own motivational speaker. Which is why, on the day that I found a cheap flight to Mexico, I invited him to join me on this trip. In the next breath, however, I focused on putting him off. I guess my urge to run away is greater than I thought.

Perhaps this will go well, and not end scarily at all. Perhaps diving is just what I need. I recall a recent conversation I had with a man named Dean Upson. Dean is a British diving instructor, working out of Malta for a dive shop. He was jovial, fast-talking. The kind of guy you'd expect to crack all the bawdiest jokes at the pub; to bring in the next round of beers, and add in two packs of pork scratchings while he's at it. But it wasn't long before I learned about the stresses behind his smiles.

Dean told me how, before he became a dive instructor, he was a corporal from 33 Engineer Regiment (EOD) – the EOD standing for Explosive Ordnance Disposal – and served with them in Afghanistan as a bomb disposal expert. During his tours, he was attached to something called a medical emergency response team (MERT); the British military's version of the flying ambulance service. As a member of the MERT, he would be among the first to respond to horrific scenes on the ground. To help a soldier burnt so badly they couldn't tell she was a woman until they noticed her bra. To treat a young man who'd been shot through the head, and take him to the hospital, where he died. To attend to the blood-covered casualties of another suicide bomber in a public place. While still on duty in Afghanistan, Dean began to show signs of suffering from post-traumatic stress disorder (PTSD). Sitting alone, with a pistol in his mouth, he had his first brush with suicide.

Dean asked for support before leaving the country; before heading home for the rest and relaxation time already due to him. *Try to recuperate there*, said support staff. *See how you feel after that.* When he arrived back to continue his tour, Dean was sent to a new area, in a move that was described to him as a 'break'. The change of scene might have helped had that new area not been Sangin, a district in Helmand Province where the Brits were undergoing relentless, bloody sieges from the Taliban. Despite the worsening of his personal issues, Dean's reluctance to leave his EOD colleagues one man down in volatile Sangin was so strong it took a painful fall, and the flare-up of an old physical injury, to finally lead him away from the front and back to the UK. This time, he spent six weeks in the military wing of a hospital, a period in which Dean said he frequently broke down, screaming and crying. He described how his requests for help with his mental health were barely acknowledged.

We hadn't been speaking for long when Dean told me he'd made four attempts on his life so far. And that he knows many more ex-servicemen who've been through similar ordeals. (Tragically, a number of them are no longer around.)

'I tried everything for the PTSD,' said Dean. 'All sorts of weird and wonderful stuff. Looking through sheets of coloured glass, meditating, even a breathing and movement programme that looked a bit like alternative dance. Some things helped more than others. I went on a residency that had mindfulness sessions, and the instructor gave us each a pebble to focus on, something to look at and meditate with. I didn't get it at all. I walked out. On the last day of the residency, I came back and the instructor asked me if I'd come to learn again. I told her, "No, I've come to give you your pebble back." She got angry with me when I said that, making out like I hadn't tried hard enough. But she didn't understand: for me, a pebble isn't something calm. I saw what pebbles can do when I was on tour. They get picked up by blasts and can cut through a person. I'd come on this course to get over my PTSD, and the instructor had given me a weapon to look at.'

Although we were talking about a disturbing topic, Dean's disposition seemed matter-of-fact, almost cheerful. But when I asked him how he got over his PTSD, the smile disappeared.

'You don't get over it,' he said. 'You deal with it.'

I thought of the things I wanted to get over. Get over and *not* have to deal with.

My chat with Dean continued. He told me that the way he now deals with PTSD – the intense anxiety, the lowness, the suicidal thoughts – is by embracing scuba. He had regularly dived before his illness and enjoyed it, even going as far as obtaining PADI's Divemaster certification – a licence that qualifies divers to supervise others in certain conditions. During his time in the Forces, he had far less time to devote to the practice. But once PTSD had set in, after desperately searching for coping strategies, a friend kitted him up, and told him to sit at the bottom of the pool. And that's what he did. Just sat there on the tiles, underwater, and breathed.

There he felt a calm he could not experience while at the surface.

'There are no triggers for me underwater,' he explained. 'No sights or sounds or smells that can set me off. Before that point I'd been living like Gollum. I felt like I couldn't engage with anything. But being in the water then was perfect. Absolute bliss.'

For Dean, diving is escapism. It's freedom. The practice keeps his mind occupied. And protects him from things like dust, loud noises, the smell of hot rubbish – everyday things that seem mundane, but which take Dean to the places where his mind most fears to go.

'Diving saved my life,' said Dean. He told me about the existence of certain therapeutic scuba programmes: scuba courses for veterans, created to make the most of diving's benefits. I spoke to a man he knows called Rob, an ex-RAF engineer whose legs were almost amputated following a motorcycling accident in the UK. His injuries were so severe he required three years of rehab in a military hospital. Though he learned to walk again, he can no longer do the sports he used to love. Apart from diving.

After his accident, Rob became a BSAC instructor (BSAC being the British Sub-Aqua Club – the UK's governing body for snorkelling and scuba). Rob now runs courses in Malta with the charity Help for Heroes. In the water, Rob told me, his legs don't hurt any more. And the amputees he's taught have had a similar experience. The diving frees them. It empowers them.

'Someone who's got no legs can still scuba dive as well as someone who's got legs,' he said. 'Someone who's got no arms can still do it. Being by the water, on the water, underwater, is very useful for them.'

He told me that some veterans join the course even though they're afraid of the sea. 'You wonder why they want to do a scuba diving course,' he laughed, 'but you persevere, and you show all the techniques. how it's safe; how things work. And they go on to enjoy it.'

Towards the end of our conversation, Rob shared a motto from his time in the military with me. It was this one: *Knowledge dispels fear.*

It makes sense, this motto. For there's the shallows, and then there's the deep. There is seeing, and not seeing. Visibility is everything. Observe the threat fully, understand, and there won't be any surprises. But mask it, blur it, leave a blank, and imagination will flood into the gaps.

Ignorance: cause.

Fear: effect.

*

Before I try for the caves, I take a detour to the island of Cozumel. There I slope quickly back into hostel life. Leaving my backpack under a roof made of straw, I go on the hunt for an escapade. I'm on the lookout for shady sights and characters; other people with fears to contend with; dark yearnings they want to fulfil. But there's no sharkish intrigue here. Just a group of smiling young people at the starts and ends of various long-term itineraries. They're polite. They talk about Europe. They try very hard to make everyone like them. I do the same, until I stop liking myself.

Alone, I walk to the sea and stand in the shallows, my trousers rolled up to my knees. The palm trees sift strong breezes. A gargantuan cruise ship is loitering in the bay, and I wonder what swims underneath it; whether, in its journey from Cuba, or around the Gulf of Mexico, this ship has passed over creatures more grotesque than itself. When I return to the hostel, a Swedish girl is packing up to go. She only arrived this afternoon, at about the same time as me, but she says this island's too boring. She wants to go back to party in Playa del Carmen. I won't be going to party in Playa del Carmen. I am tired of people, right now. Tired of postponing my immersion. Instead, tomorrow, I'll dive in the open sea. Break myself back into the water. I've heard there's a species here called the saucereye porgy. And another with the name of puddingwife. Imagine finding something called a puddingwife and being afraid.

Surely I can't be afraid. I've seen far worse than a puddingwife this past year.

Yet the following morning, I approach the prospect of diving with the usual trepidation. Liquid guts: yes. Heart fluttering: yes. Bouncy leg: uncontrollable. If a doctor opened me up right now and said my stomach was filled with live saucereye porgies, I'd believe them. I'm more or less a saucereye porgy myself. When I arrive at the dive centre, I soon learn more about the sea around here. Namely that these waters don't stay still. Not many waters do, of course. Cozumel waters, however, have their own kind of rapidity. Which means we won't be doing the usual slow-moving explore. Instead we will be drift diving: dropped in at one point, carried by strong currents across the reef, and – hopefully – collected at the end. The water will be our master.

My airways narrow further when I hear there are bull sharks in these parts. Tiger sharks, too; hunters, striped in adolescence, that can grow to more than 5 metres long, just shy of three times the length of my own body. According to certain sources, the tiger shark rivals great whites and bulls when it comes to unprovoked human attacks, though I also hear that, mostly, they hunt at night.

I must try not to think too much about bull sharks and tigers. I know that today my aim must be to focus on my diving; to endeavour to always keep close to my group and make sure I am collected with the others. What nobody wants is the same fate as the Lonergans, Eileen and Thomas, the couple from Louisiana who were left behind by their dive boat on the Great Barrier Reef. No one knew they were missing until two days later, when a bag of their belongings was spotted onboard. A message calling for help was found, but the Lonergans never were.

Perhaps Granny Codd was lucky in comparison. Perhaps the Lonergans had the worst kind of end. I can imagine few things bleaker than floating in a vast and indifferent sea, two bodies with nothing to cling to but each other. No rest. No shade. No rescue. No wonder there are so many films that exploit this fear for their audiences; the fear of being lost in the ocean; of being lost in the unknown. *Abandon Ship! The*

Reef. The Shallows. Two Came Back. Open Water. The Deep.
All of these films, and more besides, playing on the incomprehensible magnitude of water. Playing on the truth that, when removed from our fellow humans, when stripped of all we know, we are pointless. Useless nothings.

Tormenting ourselves with these kinds of thoughts is by no means a modern trend. Not for the first time, a particular section of *Moby-Dick* comes to mind – the one in which the cabin boy, Pip, is temporarily left alone in the sea and turns mad as a result: 'Now, in calm weather, to swim in the open ocean is as easy to the practised swimmer as to ride in a spring-carriage ashore. But the awful lonesomeness is intolerable. The intense concentration of self in the middle of such a heartless immensity, my God!'

Today I will be the loudest, most unmissable person onboard. Never mind being tired of people – I'll talk to everyone. If they get back aboard and it's suddenly quiet, they'll all know I'm still underwater. Whether they prefer it that way or not is something else.

On our drive to the docks, I find a useful ally in that quest. Lenny, from Toronto, is not a diver this group could forget in a hurry. His tactic is also less vocal (and thus less annoying) than my own: while everyone else is pulling on rented wetsuits, Lenny eases into his personal skinsuit, coloured the same neon green as Borat's mankini. On top of it goes a sleeveless, moss-coloured shorty (a dinky wetsuit with cut-off legs) that Lenny can't quite zip up.

'Looks like I've put on weight since last time,' he announces, chuckling. Meanwhile his suncream is spread so thickly his face looks like a ghost's. If a pea plant could be haunted, it might look something like this.

Lenny has dived in Cozumel more than ninety times, he tells me. He booked his flight for this trip with just forty-five minutes to spare before the check-in desk closed, grabbing only his dive bag and no case for extra clothes.

I like Lenny straight away. Which is fortunate because he's in my morning sub-group of recreational divers.

When we reach the mooring, Lenny leaves the speedboat first. I follow immediately after. Then the divemaster jumps in to lead the way. Down we go, fast, into the blue. There is so much blue. Reef below and to the right, then ocean stretching off for 1000 miles, no land to break it until the coast of Colombia. Right there is the prospect of losing myself, a hell of a long way to drift. But looking into that blue is not like looking at 1000 miles of oblivion. Instead it is like looking at a blank screen. Something two-dimensional. Something very separate from myself. I'm surprised I'm not more worried. This feels like rather an interesting discovery.

I still want to know how I'd react if an enormous swimming being appeared on that screen, but when nothing enormous appears I give up and pay more attention to the reef. Carried along by the current we speed above it, no opportunities to pause or linger. I breathe and am transported. The divemaster guides Lenny and me to a swim through a section of overhanging reef creating a short tunnel of marine flora – and I keep myself as steady as I can, convinced I'm going get tangled or hit the sides of it with my air cylinder. The moment I think I'm about to make it through I lightly graze my bare leg on a piece of fire coral. The skin prickles and burns. I deserve it for intruding. I'm too clumsy. Too not-fish.

The currents lead us to a group of brown garden eels that poke up like wavering fingers from the sea floor. They skittishly watch our progress, retreating into their holes when we're too close. An Atlantic stingray skims over the sand, sensing the way with its flattened snout and trailing a liquorice whip of a tail. Nothing here appears to be on the attack. This feels more like a canter through the woods than a wild safari.

Eventually we pull into a current-free patch of reef. Five metres below the surface we hover, holding a shared line, our bloodstreams decompressing so that nothing will rupture or fizz. All of us are together. I hear the engine of our boat approach.

Topside, we ride the waves to dive two. I feel unexpectedly positive, even more so when Lenny compliments my buoyancy.

'You looked calm in there,' he says. 'Very much in control.'

When my brain tries to sabotage this welcome moment of respite – *Of course you looked calm: there weren't any big fish* – I take a breath and ask Lenny to tell me more about the highlights of his job, providing tech support at a university.

'I once fixed some software right in the middle of a pig's MRI scan,' he says. 'They wouldn't have finished without me.'

It's not the kind of answer I was envisaging. Now I'm thinking about a hospital full of pig patients, staffed by pigs, pigs dressed in scrubs, pig cleaners with mops, porcine family members queuing up for piggy cappuccinos.

After orange juice and biscuits – a break to regather our strength – the pigs have vanished and we're all of us back in the water. As soon as we descend, as soon as it's too late to ask what he's doing, I notice that our divemaster is carrying a spear. I can't remember seeing that spear before. What new risk would mean he needs a spear?

There is no chance to gesture at him or work this out. The current here is faster. Life is everywhere. *Maybe the spear is for sharks.* I force myself to look up and around me. I see starfish and butterfly fish. Parrotfish smiling dopily as they munch off chunks of coral. There are small, inquisitive gobies that perch on rock ledges like lizards. Spotty, boxy specimens of smooth trunkfish, pursing their lips. Watching their shapes and colours, entranced by the way these fish interact in the water, I am quickly reduced to a pair of curious eyes, and it's hard to keep hold of my worries. Lenny catches my attention and points out a crab that's the size of his head. At the sight of the crab I feel fine, and give my green buddy an *OK* to show that I've seen it. Then I cast a glance to the blue again. The colour of it is so placid. So bright. Could this blue really be the true colour of danger? In my present state of mind it seems unlikely.

Moments later, the divemaster turns around; drifts backwards. He is forming a signal at us: a hand on his forehead, pointing straight up like a fin. I know that signal. *Shark*. He points and makes the signal again. *Shark. That way.* There's no time to panic before we're carried over a pocket of reef to where the man is pointing. And there it is. The first shark I've ever swum with. Me, the open water and a shark.

The shark is small. No longer than my leg. It is curled up on the sea floor like a cashmere scarf. A nurse shark in a hollow.

And the water is already carrying us away from it.

I keep looking back, watching out, wondering if it will come after us. But the shark doesn't stir. It is resting. I feel OK.

When I turn my face forward I'm just in time to see our divemaster lift his spear and set it in motion. The long blade charges out and tears through the middle of a lionfish. The movement is clinically lethal, an act of killing so fast that, for a brief moment, I'm sure that the fish is both dead and alive at once. In the next moment, it exists in a single state. Gone for ever. Still gripping the fish in the claw of his spear, still carried along by the current, our divemaster feels for a stowed pair of scissors, and proceeds to snip off its poisonous, vibrant quills. They float to the sea bed like feathers in our slipstream. The dead fish's eyes bulge and pop. I know that a sight like this would make me hot and sick out of the water. But right now I still feel disconnected. Absorbed, not alarmed.

The current brings us on to a giant green moray, to which the divemaster offers his just-plucked fish. The eel takes it in with one gulp. I later learn that lionfish are this region's most prevalent pests. Non-native to America and the Caribbean, they are hoovering up resources, destabilising the eco-system. These lionfish have no predators and can churn out offspring at a disconcerting rate.

We begin to ascend to the surface and I notice a commotion. I follow the divemaster's gestures and look out into the blue for the final time. There I see something amazing: a spotted eagle ray – a flattened shark with dazzling spots that is globally threatened by fishing. These rays grow up to 5 metres long, 3 metres across at the wings, and although we're quite a distance from it, maybe 30 metres, this particular one looks as if it could be large. Very large indeed. I reach for Lenny, who's studying his fins, and poke him in the arm. He turns and spots it too. The ray is swimming away from us, getting further. And, I can't believe what I'm seeing, but alongside it is a sea turtle; a hawksbill of about 1 metre long, patterned like a squat, swimming giraffe. This species is critically endangered, just a step on the chain from being extinct. But here it is. Here both of them are. Gliding through this vast wall of water, on a path through life that no one can predict.

There is not enough air left in our tanks to follow, so we breach the surface, inflate our BCD vests and float on top of the waves. Our boat is in sight, the crew beckoning. It is good to see them, but my mind is elsewhere. I can't help thinking: *One minute later and we would have missed that scene.*

At our divemaster's signal, we start to swim back to the boat. 'Wasn't that awesome?' beams Lenny as we go.

I wonder how many other creatures have been a single minute out of my sight.

'I guess you can see why I keep coming back,' Lenny croons. *How many whale sharks.*

Lenny's excitement is palpable. Clinging on to the side of the hull, hanging at the surface, I inelegantly pull off my fins and weight belt, and haul them up to the crew. I grip on to the lowest rungs of the ladder and realise that I'm excited too. Never mind what I might have missed, at last this is something I haven't. I tell myself: *I have drift-dived. I have passed over a nurse shark. I have watched a man harpoon a lionfish and feed it to a giant green moray.*

I pull myself up a few rungs towards the gunwale. The sea slaps at my thighs. *What's more*, I think, *I have actually seen a hawksbill and a spotted eagle ray.*

I am back inside the boat now. The divemaster hands out more biscuits. Lenny is chattering about the excellent free salsa classes near his hotel; how solo tourists congregate and learn all the dance moves together. It seems bizarre now that, fleetingly, under the water, Lenny, myself and the divemaster were almost entirely dependent on each other. Above the waves, however, our survival no longer relies on buddying up. Those links have already been weakened by the sun and open air. If I liked dancing classes, or thought holding hands with strangers would save my life, I might be tempted to go to salsa with Lenny. But the truth is I don't like dancing classes, or holding strangers' hands. The truth is I'd rather be alone to concentrate on the new feeling I'm experiencing: I am so much more content with myself than I was before I went into the water. I feel calm. Capable. Genuinely keen to dive again.

I start to think that if I can stay afloat and in control on a fast current, I might be able to keep my cool within a

Mexican cave system. And maybe, once I've done that, I could even keep my cool in the company of a whale shark.

Tomorrow I'll ride a catamaran to the mainland. I'll catch a bus to Tulum, base for exploring a clutch of well-known *cenotes* – submerged limestone sinkholes which dot the Yucatán peninsula; bodies of water, sacred in Mayan lore, connected as one by a mass underground river system. I'll find a responsible dive school to take me, and prove to myself that I can work through what daunts me. Soon, I will be an accomplished diver, fully prepared for all fish including whale sharks. Jackie Cousteau, they'll call me. Womanfish. I'll never panic. I'll feel no weird emotions or awkward phobias.

No fears.

Never.

Not me.

Another town, another hostel. This one serves free caipirinhas from 5 p.m. until 7 p.m. every night, which is all the incentive I need to know I'm staying in the right place. That afternoon, after skyping Max – 'Wow! You're totally nailing those fish!' – I wander the scorched Tulum streets, past large iguanas that sprawl, dozing, on the pavement, and enter another selection of kit-filled dive shops. One of them is run by female divers, a rarity as far as my experience goes, and when I mention it's my birthday tomorrow, the woman behind the desk gives me a high five. She tells me how much I'll love my 'dirty thirties'.

'So how are you going to celebrate?' she asks. I can do a day of three dives in local cenotes, or try out a dive with a school of adult bull sharks. If I'm here for more than one day, she says, I could book myself on to both.

Bull sharks *and* cenotes? I duck out of the shop to check my bank balance. The amount behind the scratched ATM glass says the option of both is off. I think about those bull sharks; their powerful jaws, their movement, their constant appetites. Then I think about the alternative: darkness, enclosure, stillness. I try to work out which option I fear the most. Which I should aim to confront.

I return to the high-fiving woman and book the cave dives. Three of them, one for each decade I've lived so far. I wonder whether, if I keep diving, I'll be able to make it all the way through my fourth.

As I sign the relevant waivers, I feel my Cozumel confidence trickle away.

The Pit is the deepest cenote in the state of Quintana Roo, and extends underground by some 119 metres. Surrounded by dusty jungle, it's part of the subterranean system of Dos Ojos (translation: Two Eyes). At the bottom of the shallower main chamber, I hear, ancient human and animal remains can be seen. Sacrificial fragments, the significance of which is long-forgotten, they are shrouded by mists of hydrogen sulphide. If all goes according to plan, I won't be getting deep enough to see them for myself.

We arrive at the site just before 10 a.m. and park the truck as an early diver enters The Pit with his buddy. The taste of a birthday-cake breakfast is already souring on my lips. Our instructor, Xanath, wants to enter the water with us early too, before the rest of the crowds arrive to join.

The route to the cave leads us via a wooden platform with sheer scaffolded stairways. It looks like part of a film set, a rickety prop from *Indiana Jones and the Temple of Doom*. Clambering down the steps in heavy gear, I find it hard to believe that, within this part-concealed pond, a huge cave chamber waits to be explored. Harder to believe that, in a few moments, I'll be one of the divers to explore it; that this is where my focus on fear has taken me.

The cavern looks suitably creepy and forbidding. Its mouth seems to open at our approach: a shark's mouth that invites me to look deeper. *Here I am*, it says. And then: *Beware*.

From these well-worn planks, it's just a short leap into the water. I glance around at my fellow divers, a group of four smiling people, all keen to crack on. It is time for us to descend. I close my eyes and make the jump. The cenote's waters close over my head, then pop me back up, floating. The others from my group drop like stones, splashing down beside me. As we prepare to dive, I peer through my mask, through the dark surface, and take in the scene below us. Tranquil, bottomless blue. Clustering spears of sunlight. A slightly hazy disturbance in the water. That, announces Xanath, is the halocline: the point at which the cenote's freshwater layer meets the saline. We're going to pass through it on our way down, she says, and, if we're lucky, our early dive will mean it has not grown thick from diver disturbance. If we're unlucky there will be metres of blurred, confusing water to push through. It's my birthday. My first ever cave dive. I'd appreciate some good luck.

Xanath has given us each a torch, and a numbered position we need to remain in. I am Diver Number Three behind her. Diver Three, doing three dives, on my thirtieth. I'm not sure what this means in terms of omens.

Together we take the plunge and stay in formation. We are travelling to our dive's deepest point first, which means passing through the halocline right off the bat. And although I've just been briefed about its presence, the effect of it still takes me by surprise. My eyes scramble to adjust to the unadjustable: smeared vision in every direction; people and walls reduced to incomprehensible globs. My mind kicks in, reminding me that this is was supposed to happen. And suddenly we're through to the other side.

When I spoke to Vas in James Deane's shop, he described how the boundless clarity of cenotes created a dive experience which felt to him like flying. To me it is more like falling. Several times I throw my arms into the nothingness, unsure whether I'm buoyant or sinking down. No matter how it moves against my skin, the still water looks like air. The cave walls, meanwhile, seem far away and offer no support. I feel destabilised. I feel unnerved. But at the same time the cenote is beguiling. Visibility tops 60 metres. The skeleton of a tree claws through the water. We navigate over dead branches, glimpsing torchlights way beneath us through the milky, acidic fog. Down there are divers far braver – far more advanced – than I am. Perhaps more reckless too. In the distance a single eel threads through the water, the only form of non-human life I see.

Leaving our own dive's lowest point, we journey towards the enclosed roof of the cavern, circling in our slow line of five explorers. As I look up to a near section of overhang I suddenly notice inverse pools of stars, where pockets of air are trapped beneath the rocks. These upside-down pools have an eerie halo. They play optical tricks. On the approach, they look like spilt oil. Dark, yet iridescent and alive. Then they become burnt mirrors that reflect back, with an orange hue, the clarity of the water. The closer I get, the more this sheen fades, until finally, from a point directly beneath them, I can see right through to the stone ceiling above.

My fears shrink in the presence of pools like these. They exist, I exist, and all I feel is a strong desire to watch them. In time, our gentle rotations take us back up through the halocline – another few seconds of blurring – and then, once again, we're at the surface, unscathed. I am ecstatic.

One cave down. Two more to go.

It's a short ride over dirt roads to reach our second set of dive sites at Dos Ojos, two spots known as The Barbie Line and The Bat Cave. The vibe here is quite different to The Pit. The car park is almost full. Big groups of children cluster in life vests, and coaches unload their riders in groups of thirty or more. My group and I snack on corn crisps and lukewarm tamales, leaning against the open boot of the truck. Everyone's in high spirits. Especially me. It's my birthday and everyone knows it. Even the strangers I meet on my way to the toilet.

'I'm thirty today.'

'I'm smiling because it's my birthday.'

'Just off on some birthday cave dives.'

As the time for our car park break counts down, I feel my insides slither, and am obliged to start using this flush of hyperactivity to mask a more familiar flush (less welcome) of apprehension. The unknown is unsettling me, yet again. For the next two dives will be quite different to the first, presenting their own sets of risks. Unlike The Pit, they will not be in wide, open spaces with a natural light supply, but underwater tunnels, jagged and largely sunless – the kind of environments Vas and Mungo know well, but I do not. While down, we will have to follow a line that's laid out in the water. And, Xanath explains to us, we will have to follow it closely. To protect both ourselves and the delicate walls of the cave, we need to remain a metre above the line the whole way through; laying our torsos flat in the water, our calves raised behind us at right angles; holding a pose not unlike that of freefalling skydivers. Float too high and we'll hurt ourselves on the rock. Float too low and we might be caught by the line. Lose the line altogether and we could be lost too. On which note, we also need to use our torches. Without them we might not be able to see what's in front of us.

Kitted up, our tamales finished, we waddle to the deck beside the cave entrance, where a group of Chinese children are floating in vests, masks and snorkels, delighted by the luminous blue of the water. Their antics look fun but superficial, and suddenly I have an urge to leave the noise behind. *Let's get this over with.* We jump in and sink beneath the snorkellers, gaining a shark's-eye view of kicking legs and commotion. Breathing steadily, we make our way to the start of The Barbie Line, keeping our respective places as we did in The Pit. No overtaking. No swimming in pairs. The line is the line, and that's it.

This is not a dive for anyone claustrophobic. Wax-like stalagmites grow beneath us. Dark walls encroach on the water. In some of the tunnels, boulders crowd the floor. Occasional breaks in the roof permit snatches of light, but the torch is my constant eye and I fix it wherever I can. This time there's not even an eel to give a fleeting impression of life. Instead we pass the sight of a nude Barbie doll caught in the mouth of a toy crocodile – the crude plastic formation installed by Nobody-Knows-Who, and which gives this route its name. As we leave these childish characters behind, I wonder if this cenote could contain any real crocodiles. Surely not. Hopefully not.

My torch flickers. As the stone walls converge around us, my control, my buoyancy, seem to be OK. Until we slow down. Then I start to lose it. There is a blockage ahead. Diver One is rising up too high. But his wife, Diver Two, sees it happen. She grabs his ankle and pulls him back down. Xanath doesn't notice. We know that she probably won't unless we signal her, shaking at her back with the strobes of our lights, but no one wants to be the first to do it. Meanwhile, in the absence of forward motion, I start to sink. I shoot more air into my BCD, but in my haste I add too much. Now I, too, am rising slowly away from the line, on my way to a ceiling of crags. I'm going to be punctured. Stabbed in the back of the skull by the roof. Flapping my hands and fumbling, I eventually manage to locate the button I need, and let out the excess air just in time, all too aware that Diver Four is behind me, watching me flail; that my messy movements will hamper his own progress. I'm also aware that the gap between us and the front-runners is widening.

Slow breaths, Georgie. Just follow the line.

I can see why a diver like Mungo would want to go solo. I can also see how things can go so badly wrong. Our maximum depth on this line is just shy of 8 metres. We don't have to contend with deep pressures, and the line is already laid for us. But still we're having difficulties and, for much of the route, are unable to reach open air. I pacify myself with the thought that hundreds, possibly thousands, of divers with limited cave experience have traced this well-marked route without fatalities. Or at least, if there have been deaths here, I couldn't find any word of them online.

After fifty minutes of trailing rope, we come back into full daylight, where another batch of snorkellers' legs paddles furiously. We have made it through The Barbie Line's clutches intact, and I feel stronger again. Now there is just one dive left. This will be to The Bat Cave, the other well-known cave dive of Dos Ojos. The tunnels will be narrower. Darker. The way will be more constricted. But I think it will be something I can do. I just have to breathe slowly. To move gently. To keep an eye on the air I'm using. To stay in my place. I have a place.

This time in the water, I reassure myself that the present moment is all that matters. That and the gauge. The breaths.

The line. I accept that I am going into darkness. Shining
a light towards the unknown. And while the thought of
this unknown may be appalling, at least it's a direction I
can aim for.

In fixing on to this unknown, I see underwater fossils.
Mayan gobies. A cavern filled with furry bats, hanging like
giant flies in a stalactite web. As we continue along the route,
my torch dies and my pupils dilate to black holes. I cannot
signal to the others. I am guided by their lights. Beyond
them the world is murky; near-black. There is no escape but
what comes from moving forward. So we swim. Through
chambers. Past deathly corridors. Over tumours of calcified
rock. My anxiety does not take over. I can't afford to let it. I
know I must focus on my cavernous surroundings. Focus on
the belly of the giant. Its innards offer no comfort but they
are captivating nonetheless. Gradually I realise I'm enjoying
the sensation of veering past the black nooks and through the
crannies. I am the captain of my movements. I control the
water, and the water does not control me. *Look at me, gobies,*
I'm thinking. *I am one of you. I am a fish.*

I follow the line to the end without any more problems, no
further incidents to challenge my newfound hubris. In spite
of my lack of training, in spite of my own panic tendencies, a
third roll of the dice has come up in my favour. I have dived
through a system of Mexican cave tunnels, in part without a
fully functioning torch, *and I survived.*

The caves have switched off my panic brain. For better or
worse, I feel ready to go deeper.

11

Here Be Monsters

'You're not a fish.'

DIVE INSTRUMENTS,
PADI OPEN WATER MANUAL, 1999–2007

It's a huge relief to be back in London, a feeling I haven't experienced in this city for a while. Somehow, life seems to be stabilising. I am offered a side-job writing copy for a friend's company, and will soon give up my shifts at the clinic to dedicate more of my time to it. I've also found a cheap one-bed annexe to live in, away from the grime and hubbub, away from my old flat, sheltered on three sides by trees. This part of the city doesn't feel like London. I'm five minutes' walk from the nearest outdoor swimming pool, and go there with Max after work. We punch our way through the lengths until we're knackered. It feels good to be swimming again. And even though the waters here are fishless, I feel like I'm making progress.

Once I'm settled in my new place and enjoying my new routine, I start a course called *Coping with Difficult Emotions.* It sounds like the kind of course everyone needs – especially when they're planning to smite a phobia. Or use that phobia to deal with something else.

In a group of ten, we are invited to share our difficult emotions. Some come out easier than others. My disappointment at Ted. My fears that I'm just not good enough; that I have achieved nothing, and never will; that the people I love will all leave me through death, or otherwise. I say all I feel able to say, then the next person takes their turn.

Together, we discuss how the brain works. We're told about neural pathways – how they are formed and can be broken. How easy it is to get caught up in cycles. How changing the way we think and feel can come by way of small, repeated alterations in our behaviour. We are also encouraged to download an app of spoken meditations. I try to sit through ten minutes of these every day. When Max stays over he joins in, then falls asleep before they're done. Upright, awake, beside him, I feel worthy. Meditation is surely a wholesome pastime. The kind of pastime a calm person would do. And sometimes, in brief flashes, even without an air tank, I feel calm.

The course leads me through summer. In the third of our weekly sessions, the therapist invites us to 'take in the good'. This means that, to help rewire our brains, we should relive positive memories four times every day; kind words someone has said to us; an uplifting experience; a special meal.

He asks us to visualise ourselves in our favourite place. We close our eyes and to my surprise I'm floating in the sea. On the shore sit Granny, my mum and her dog. I feel the salt water drift across my arms; nuzzle its way along the length of my back. The smell of smoked charcoal coats the air – barbecued sunshine. There are no fears in this vision. No worries of what lies beneath. Just me, the sea and my family, sitting on the sand, keeping an eye out to check I don't drift away. It's as if my phobia doesn't exist. As if my plan to cure it is really working.

I walk home after the session as if on a cloud. I am positive. I'm getting better. More aware, and in control of my emotions. Then that night I dream that I'm watching a fish in a tank. For a while the fish seems content. But soon, as I look, its shining eyes start to bulge. In a matter of moments both of them burst, leaving two pitiful hollows in their place. I can do nothing.

When I'm fully awake and breathing normally, I sit up and download a special exercise for anxiety. The voice on the app suggests I choose a person that my mindfulness could help, someone who might benefit from my calmer state of mind. The voice has asked me to do this before, and I've picked Mum or Max. Now the person that comes to mind is not a person at all. It is a whale shark.

Maybe the big fish is not my nemesis. Maybe death is not my nemesis. Maybe my *only* nemesis is the unknown, and all I need do is learn how to approach it.

Only, that raises a substantial question: how can I overcome a fear of the unknown when I'll never be able to know it? If the unknown is the author of my fears, the ocean could be its bestseller. The book of the sea is full of gargantuan blanks, of things no one can grasp: speculations that turn appalling under the black magic of our nerves.

In 2012, the film director James Cameron became only the third human to look straight into the deepest known part of the ocean – an area in the Mariana Trench known as the Challenger Deep, which is located about 6.7 miles down in the western Pacific, near Guam – and observe what was around him. Seven years later, a retired Texan naval officer, Victor Vescovo, would complete a similar mission, reaching an even deeper spot in the trench with his submarine, *Limiting Factor*. The *first* two humans to manage the feat, Jacques Piccard and Dom Walsh, did so together, in 1960. But their vessel threw up so much sediment on impact they saw even less than they'd planned.

With a team of ambitious technicians, and a budget of $35,000 a day, James Cameron closed a gap of fifty-two years by creating a racing-green submersible robust enough to withstand more than seven tonnes of pressure per square inch. If we could hold the weight of an adult blue whale in our palms, we'd have some idea of what those numbers mean. We'd also no longer have palms. Crushed into their smallest atomic components, those palms might never have existed.

The feature-length movie of James Cameron's voyage, *Deepsea Challenge*, puts it another way: down at the very deepest depths, the strength of water pressure is so powerful that a leak in the sub could cut a man in half.

To help mitigate a fear of the deep, you can now look, via a TV screen, into the deepest known part of the sea. Peering past James Cameron's shoulder, you can gaze onto the Mariana Trench, a place so deep Mount Everest would fit at the bottom with room for more than one full vertical mile of water between its peak and the sea's surface.

This region, the deepest layer of the ocean, is known as the hadopelagic, or hadal zone. It is named after Hades, Greek god of the underworld. Sunlight can't reach it. Divers can't reach it. James Cameron and Victor Vescovo have. But the chances are you won't reach it for yourself. Unless you watch their footage.

If you do choose to do that, you'll see what they have seen. The desolate nothingness. The sand, or whatever substance it is that can still hold its shape at that depth. Not to mention the impenetrable blackness outside their vessels' light supplies.

On screen, before the credits to *Deepsea Challenge* start rolling, Cameron includes a short note to his viewers. The note reports that, in all the deep-sea trenches of the world, *an area the size of North America remains as yet undiscovered.* I cannot get my head around that statement. I've tried. I just can't. And it seems likely that, even if I could, I would have a reaction like the woman in Douglas Adams' *The Restaurant at the End of the Universe*, who is plugged into her husband's invention, the Total Perspective Vortex:

> [Into] one end he plugged the whole of reality as extrapolated from a piece of fairy cake, and into the other end he plugged his wife: so that when he turned it on she saw in one instant the whole infinity of creation and herself in relation to it.

The shock of the vision annihilates her brain.

How does anyone cope with the concept of all those unknowns, I wonder. How can I?

Dr Jon Copley is a bathynaut, a person who uses submersible vehicles, such as bathyspheres or bathyscaphes, to see what exactly is happening in our deep oceans. According to his website, he is the first Brit to have gone as deep as he has gone – to a depth of 3.1 miles, to be precise; to the deep-sea thermal vents of the Cayman Trough.

You might think that a scientist doing this work would harbour, and cultivate, a thoroughly pragmatic attitude, free from fear and phobia. But apparently that is not the case. In response to a message I send him, Jon writes: 'I was scared of the water as a child and learned to swim quite late. I still get anxious if I'm in the water at the surface of the ocean, not really being able to see what's in the void below. But put me in a sub, diving to a previously unseen ocean floor, and that anxiety vanishes.'

Fear at the surface seems to be a common diving trait. It's a boost to know I'm not alone. And that, for those who show willing, the departure from what's known can lead to some spellbinding places.

For days before I speak to Jon Copley in person, I tell anyone who'll listen that I'm going to meet a bathynaut. 'An actual real-life bathynaut,' I say.

Everyone who hears this looks at me blankly.

'What's a bathynaut?' they say. All except for a university friend, who thinks for a moment about what I said, and answers: 'Is that like an astronaut, but for the bath?'

'Yes,' I tell her. 'Exactly.'

On the day that Jon and I meet, conditions are the opposite of the bathynaut's usual climate. It's bright. Dry. Hot. Spacious. And people are everywhere. While I wait, I fan my reddening face with the copy of *Moby-Dick* I've been rereading. When I open it up I chance on a line with shades of the motto I heard from Rob, the Help for Heroes diver: 'Ignorance is the parent of fear,' says Ishmael. I'm too agitated about my meeting to read anything more.

Moments later, Jon arrives in a casual outfit of shorts and wrap-around sunnies. A satchel is over his shoulder. He is instantly recognisable from his website and online videos (sample: 'There's no longer any part of the deep ocean that's inaccessible to us if we can find the will to go there.') I look at the people around us. *You don't know*, I think. *This man has been to the depths of the oceans, he's seen things that the rest of us can't even imagine. And all you're doing is knocking back the beers.*

Then I wonder how many bathynauts *I've* passed without ever knowing they were bathynauts. I wonder how many bathynauts there *are*. This pondering shapes my first question to Jon. He smiles and says it's hard to know. Depends on how you define it. Since the deep sea technically starts at 200 metres, there must be thousands, if not tens of thousands, of bathynauts.

'But bathynauts who've gone *very* deep,' Jon adds, 'to the abyssal and hadal zones of the sea, for example . . . Well, there really aren't many of those.'

I can feel myself getting more worked up. I know I should keep my cool, but I don't think I can. Because now Jon is telling me how it feels to enter the realm of the deep and unknown sea, a place not meant for humans, where nightmares have all the space they need to grow huge. Later, when I play back the recording of our conversation, I hear myself gasp at least once per sentence he speaks. *Shut up*, I think then. *Let the bathynaut talk.*

'The deep sea is so exciting when we're there,' Jon says. 'We ignore the cold and the cramp. You're aware of the pressure. The sub creaks and groans. But as long as the pilot and engineer with you aren't looking worried, you're not worried.'

I imagine the world of the bathysphere as a floating metal coffin, constantly fighting the forces that want it to come to an eternal rest. Does being a bathynaut make Jon think about death? About being eaten by gigantic sharks? About being sliced in two by pressurised leaks?

'There've been some tense moments,' he admits. 'But minor leaks are actually not that unusual, depending on the sub. Because you're in a sphere – which is the best shape for resisting pressure evenly from all sides – there are always things going through the hull, and in some cases these can be weak points. Often they *need* high pressure for the seals to really close tight. So for the first hundred metres they might leak a little.'

He sees me staring aghast.

'What you do whenever you see water in a sub,' he says, 'is you dip your finger in and taste it. If it's fresh, it's just condensation. If it's salty, probably mention it . . . ' I am still staring aghast. 'On the other hand,' he continues, 'fire is scary, because you're in such a small space that the atmosphere can go toxic *very* rapidly. It doesn't take much plastic smoke – you don't even actually need a fire with flames – to have a real problem in that environment. So that's a worry.'

Jon tells me about a time he was in a sub, and plastic smoke started filling up the interior. He and the crew were on the verge of putting on their oxygen masks, all thinking about aborting the dive, when they found the source of the problem and unplugged it.

Maybe all you need in life to deal with unknowns is a confident engineer. Except there are some things that even the best engineers can't tackle. Like the things *outside* technology; the creatures existing around the sub, way down in the depths. Those fearsome deep sea sharks I'm imagining, for instance – all the more fearsome because I know nothing about them. Dr Copley could be the first to see any number of terrifying creatures when he dives. The bogeymen under the bed. Their black mouths and glassy eyes. I move to the edge of my chair.

'You do have these odd moments when you think about where you are,' Jon says. 'A lot of the time you're really busy. You're the only scientist in the sub at the time, you've got a shopping list for everybody and your time is limited – by battery power, usually, because we're using the lights and the thrusters and arms . . .

'Occasionally you'll have to set up an instrument to make a measurement and it'll take five minutes, and then you suddenly have time to think about where you are to look out of the porthole, just to take it in. And that's when these things kind of hit you. Not so much the fear but just the— ' Jon stops himself. 'Well, no that does creep in actually. You become aware that you're in this tiny little pool of light that you can see, and then there's just darkness for hundreds of miles in every direction.' Jon laughs.

Despite the heat I have goose pimples.

'Also,' he continues, 'you're in this bubble of air and comparative warmth and so on, and outside it's cold, it's crushing pressure.'

He describes the time he looked out of the window to see

a chimaera, a species also sometimes known as a spook fish. They're closely related to sharks and rays.

'It's a bit of a Frankenstein's monster-looking thing,' says Jon. 'Like bits of other fish stitched together, with lines on its body that look like monster stitching.' When he saw one it was hanging outside his porthole and seemed to be contemplating him with its giant obsidian eye. 'And I suddenly thought, *Hang on. We're probably about a metre apart from each other* – and yet we were *worlds* apart from each other.'

Jon admits that all he sees are the creatures who come to the sub's light. He doesn't see the secret things that lurk back in the darkness; who hide from, or flee, his submersible. What he calls, *à la* Donald Rumsfeld, 'the known and unknown unknowns.'

The known knowns are intimidating enough. Out there in the depths are colossal squid. Male angler fish that latch on to their larger, light-dangling female partners, fusing with them as parasites, exchanging sperm for nutrients. There are goblin sharks with protruding gums; angular razor teeth tailor-made to impale. Even megamouth sharks – the smallest known shark in the trio of filter feeders that includes basking sharks and whale sharks – could be out there at 200 metres or more. At the latest count, only ninety-nine megamouth specimens had ever been sighted in the whole recorded history of man. *Ninety-nine.*

As for the unknown unknowns – naturally, one never knows when they might appear. In a deep-sea expedition to Puerto Rico in 2015, America's National Oceanic and Atmospheric Administration (NOAA) captured footage of several creatures that have never been seen before, and it was by no means the only expedition to do so that year. That March, the World Register of Marine Species revealed that scientists had discovered 1451 new ocean species in just twelve months. More are being found all the time. Such as the foot-long ruby seadragon, a ribbed, nymph-like creature not unlike a seahorse, which was first filmed alive in 2016 off the coast of Western Australia; such as a hydromedusa jellyfish, with luminous yellow gonads; deep-sea 'mirrorbellies' which produce light in their rectums and transmit it along their scales; a 3-metre long arapaima in Guyana that relies on inhaling surface air to live.

According to statistics from the NOAA, although two-thirds of the Earth's surface is covered by oceans, less than 5 per cent of this has been explored. There could be armies of gigantic fish down there for all we know: mutant, hardcore fish who shun the light.

I ask Jon about the creatures he has discovered on his own expeditions.

'Actually I've got some with me,' he announces, eyes a-glint. He reaches into his satchel and rummages, pulling out two clear blocks of resin. Each one contains something strange and dead at its core.

'This is the Hoff crab,' says Jon, pointing at a small, pinkish crustacean. His team found it in the Antarctic and pulled up specimens from 2500 metres below their ship. Immediately he knew he'd come across something different and new. How? Because crabs can't do cold temperatures.

The Hoff crab lives around deep thermal vents on the ocean floor. 'They're a bit like those monkeys in Japan,' Jon says, 'basking around hot springs.' Not unlike a monkey – or indeed, its *Baywatch* namesake – the crab has what look like little brown hairs sprouting out of its exoskeleton.

Trapped, dead, in the resin, the crab has lost any power it might have had in life to be frightening. I turn its resinous block over and over in my fingers. After a moment of quiet awe, I lay the Hoff crab down. I feel like I've met an alien. I point to the second block of resin.

'What's that?' I ask Jon.

'That,' he says, 'is a scaly foot snail.' He slides it across the table. As I peer at this gungy brown snail in clear plastic, I notice something resembling iron filings where a slimy mucus foot would normally be, like something from a biology poster drawn by a steampunk fanatic.

'It's covered in scaly metal plates,' Jon explains, 'made of two types of iron mineral.' The shell, it transpires, is also made partly from iron, and has the amazing power to self-heal. The creature has evolved, Jon believes, to deal with the toxic fluids of thermal vents. Now scientists are studying how it is put together to improve the way they craft life-saving structures like bicycle helmets. Soon, Jon says, he would like to explore deep-sea vents in the Atlantic, which may unlock clues to learning how proteins change their structure in diseases like cystic fibrosis and Alzheimer's.

These all seem like understandable reasons to dive in hostile conditions; important motivators to overcome fear. Jon also assures me the risks of death are statistically very small. Whereas I've imagined a sea bed littered with crushed subs and torn explorers, Jon can recall only one fatal accident since this form of exploration began in the 1930s. The accident had nothing to do with darkness, sharks or pressure. Instead, in 1973, two divers perished when their vehicle was tangled in a wreck. They died before they were rescued because the carbon dioxide scrubber in their compartment – a piece of equipment clearing the air of toxic CO_2 build-up – malfunctioned in the unexpected cold. They were, effectively, poisoned by their own breaths. (The designer who built the sub was doubly punished: one of the divers killed was his own son.)

As he mentioned in his first email to me, it's the surface of the sea that Jon finds unnerving – those times when he can't see what is underneath him. He talks about a now-banned practice on scientific vessels, something known as the 'swim call'. It formed part of his earliest expeditions to the Pacific, the aim being to give those aboard a chance to refresh in the sea. As Jon explains the details, again I think of Melville's cabin boy, Pip, turned irreversibly mad by the sight of a seemingly limitless ocean.

'You are way offshore,' says Jon, 'and the water is 3000 metres deep beneath you. You all jump off the back of the ship, and the ship steams away and it leaves you there and suddenly you're aware of how tiny you are. There's this vast void beneath you and everybody starts behaving like Antarctic penguins: you're all trying to get in the middle; no one wants to be on the outside.' Swim calls were stopped after someone on a different ship, in a different sea, was attacked by a shark. 'There are oceanic whitetips if you're in the right part of the world,' he says. 'They often follow under the shape of the boat.'

I ask Jon if he is afraid of big fish, as I am. He shakes his head. Goes as far as saying he would love to swim with great whites because he so admires the way they've adapted to what's around them: their heightened senses, their streamlined shapes, their behaviour; all the things that make them an efficient part of the food chain. It's flying in planes that really frightens Jon Copley. Or James Cameron's 1986 sci-fi *Aliens*. In a deep-sea sub, on the other hand, Jon knows and trusts the crew. All have spent a long time engaged in the planning. Plus if everything goes wrong and only he's left alive, he knows the right button to press to send the sub (and himself) back to surface.

It still sounds pretty risky to me, and I ask him if there's not a better way to do it, a way which involves less danger to those taking part. Jon admits that technological advances have made deep-sea robots a very useful tool in his research. But, he says, while those robotic subs can do an excellent job down there, it is when humans enter the sea *themselves* that the real revelations arise: 'It gives you a new perspective. Being in a sub has actually informed my research. I've noticed patterns and things. I think there's room for both.'

Makes sense, I think. Not once has it crossed my mind to find a cure for my phobia by sending down a GoPro on a stick. I want that sense of perspective for myself.

More than ninety minutes after our conversation began, Jon is preparing to catch his train home, and my legs have formed a sweat patch on the chair. All Jon has let me buy him is a single, tiny bottle of Birra Moretti. In exchange he's shared some excellent tips on how to control my fears of the unknown. These are imperative tricks for his line of work, for 'fear would be a distraction', he says, and the gateway to various dangers. Panic when the fire alarm goes off, for example, and you might not perform the right drill to sort things out. Keeping busy is his top solution – using step-by-step processes to retain a sense of focus in every event. And that's not the only thing I've picked up from Jon. I've also learned about mindset. It's clear that this man does not see terror in the world's unknown places. Instead he sees millions of cubic miles for learning, a vast space for respect and wonder, rather than death and doom.

Studiously learning more about all aspects of my fear seems like the most promising way to banish my ignorance, so I create two lists in an effort to pinpoint the issues. On one list, my Granny Codd-themed list, is:

- Pain
- Death
- Regret
- Decay

On the other list are the fish-related things; things that could happen to me while I'm aiming for whale sharks:

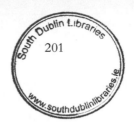
- Getting narc'd
- Contracting the bends
- Being pushed down by a 'playful' shark
- Being swallowed

Just looking at the Granny-based options makes me feel physically sick, so I fold it up and concentrate on the other one. (*'Left wrist hurting, Georgina? I'll stamp on the right.'*) Pain and dead bodies factor here too, though on this list they feel more manageable. I consider each of the fish fears again, and start to work out what I need to do to mitigate each one. I feel like I need to know more – face more and practise calmness – before I can head for the big things again. It feels mad to go straight to the whale shark.

I recognise that I'm stalling. It makes sense: my phobic instincts doing their utmost to sabotage this process. But, conveniently, rationally, it also makes sense not to risk a panic attack as a whale shark shunts towards me. Which is why, while I build up my funds again – money I earn by writing ever more marketing material – I make plans to understand narcosis better, to track down people who've had the bends, and, of course, to find people who really know the truth about the biggest fish in the ocean. That ought to keep me busy. That ought to keep my sense of purpose high.

Never mind the voice in the background that says: *You can't make this project last for ever. Sooner or later you'll meet the shark. And then what will you do?*

Working from home frees up time to pursue this next phase of my mission. In the couple of hours I would have spent commuting to the clinic every day, I now send out emails to new contacts, to friends of friends, to specialists. I want them to tell me all they know, so I can know it all. The key to understanding the ocean's unknowns, I suspect, lies within the minds of other people. People braver and more experienced than me.

But despite my doing my utmost to avoid it, on some days, the more difficult days, I'm reminded of what life can feel like without focus. These are the days when I wait for replies and contact, but nothing comes. When a freelancing brief is delayed. When Max is seeing his mates and can't stay over. When I call my friends but they're all too busy to talk. These sorts of days aren't pleasant. I try to be calm and stay in the moment – like I've been taught to do on my *Difficult Emotions* course – but can't reach the soothing, childhood sea in my head. There are no restful beach scenes with Granny, Mum and the dog on days like this.

I try to get on regardless. I shower, dress, eat toast with peanut butter. I turn on my meditation app and listen to the measured voice on my phone. The voice tells me things like, by making other people happy, I will be happy myself. I sit at my desk, close my eyes and immediately see my grandmother's body. I want to push the image away. I should probably bring it close. Only bringing Granny Codd closer like this feels unbearable.

I hear the voice of Alex, the teccie whose student drowned in front of him. I remember him saying, 'In some ways it's almost like, now it's happened, it's not such a huge fear in a weird sort of way – once it actually happens you're like, *Oh right*. You know? Life goes on.'

I hear the voice of Mandi. I remember her saying, 'I know that if I make myself sit with the panic, eventually I'll feel fine.'

And now there is also Jon Copley's way to think of: *prepare, look, learn*.

I need to become less afraid of death. I cannot keep avoiding it.

One morning, before I start sending a new round of emails, I search the web for pictures of dead bodies. More specifically,

I search for victims of drowning. Max comes in from the bathroom, about to say goodbye for the day and wish me luck. When he looks over my shoulder, he sees a graphic photograph of a dead man laid out, face up, on a patch of dirt. The man's tongue is engorged and lolling out over his teeth. There are large tracts of purple skin over his neck and bare chest, as if he has been spattered with red wine. I scroll through more thumbnail images and see a body floating in a brown river. The body is wearing its clothes but has no head. There are maggots using its neck stump as an edible dinghy, working through the remaining flesh as they go. Max puts his hand on mine and leads me away from my chair.

'What's wrong?' he says.

'I'm not sure,' I say. 'I'm researching.'

Max looks straight at me. The veins beneath his eyes are porcelain blue. They are so fragile, so close to the surface. I never noticed how shallow his blood was there. He glances past where I'm sitting, at the rows of dead people exposed on my computer.

'Maybe you should have a break,' he says. 'Would a swim make you feel better?'

'I'm not sure,' I say again.

Not long after that, I take a few days off. One of the recent emails I sent was to a man in Dorset named Mike. Mike heads up dive excursions beneath Swanage Pier and will help keep my PADI training fresh without me needing a drysuit. Swanage Pier is a bus ride away from my mum's house, so I combine the trip with an overdue visit to see her. There will be no whale sharks today; no extreme depths, or narcosis. Just gentle exploration.

It used to be that Mum and I would come to Swanage with Granny and drink hot chocolate. This time I come alone. I half-hope that the excursion will help me reclaim the town; help me to acclimatise to her absence. As it happens, when the bus pulls in, thoughts of Granny Codd are pushed from my mind by the sudden, very real fear that, in the five-and-a-half months since Mexico, I've forgotten how to dive.

On arrival Mike sees my worry and gives me a quick refresher – the set-up, the signals, the checks.

'Right,' I say when he's finished. 'I think I've got it.'

'You'll be fine,' he says. 'Just stay close to me. OK?'

'OK,' I say.

We dive the pier, our first dive of two, and instantly I'm amazed by what we can see at just 5 metres' depth. The elegant sea grasses, lushly swaying. The cloisters of sunlight and angular shadows. The rich mauve seaweeds which sprout from the sand like heather. If Egypt's Blue Hole is the Divers' Cemetery, the underneath of Swanage Pier must be the Divers' Playgroup. Everything looks soft, made hazy by good old-fashioned British visibility. Sponges roll and bounce. Drowning, death and panic seem so far away.

Mike beckons me towards a thick strut of the pier and points at a hole in the wood. I watch, curious, as he picks up a small pebble from the sea bed, then places it carefully inside the hole. A few seconds later a small fish with weed-like growths on its head emerges with the pebble in its mouth and spits it out at us. Its face is the perfect expression of indignance. This is a tompot blenny, I learn later, a species known for its distinctive, inquisitive character.

At the start of our second dive, the first sign of wildlife I see is what appears to be a saltwater lobster riding a sleek and dappled fish – most likely a wrasse. *A lobster riding a wrasse.* As if the lobster – small, dark purple, wearing its full armour – is on its way to a jousting tournament. I feel as if I've dropped into the pages of a comic book. I cannot work out what I'm seeing. I cannot believe it is real. Did the lobster fall on to the wrasse? Or did it somehow mount its fishy steed on purpose? Both scenarios seem so implausible. My brain is boggled. I try to get Mike's attention, but by the time I do the unlikely duo has galloped out of sight.

We coast over the seabed, circling the pier. Rugby-ball-sized spider crabs stand in the weeds, threatening us with segmented orange claws. The effect is of a group of knobbly men uselessly shaking their fists. There's enough distance between us to know they can't reach. And besides I'm in my mask again, hiding behind my screen.

I feel big. Safe.

I feel like I'm on the right track.

After the dive, when I'm out of my wetsuit and dressed, I'm glad to find Mum waiting for me in town, her Jack Russell terrier pulling at his lead. Damp hair is pressed to my forehead. The skin around my eyes is red, indented by the tightness of my mask. Apologising for my appearance, I give her a hug and adjust the bag of swimming gear on my shoulders. Everything feels much heavier on land. Everything *is* much heavier.

'Want to go home?' Mum asks me.

I contemplate having a nap in my childhood bedroom. Switching off my thoughts for the afternoon.

'Yes, please,' I say. 'That'd be great.'

We walk to her car and the dog skips ahead, his paws scudding excitedly over the beach. I watch the beckoning waves beside him, then glance at the high street and stop.

'Fancy a hot chocolate first?'

'Good idea,' says Mum. 'Granny would approve.'

Before I can take a breath my eyes start stinging.

'If I hadn't . . . ' I begin to say.

'If she hadn't . . . ' I try again. But my insides are too knotted to finish the sentence.

12

Mounting Pressure

'If you wait until you feel discomfort you may not be able to equalize . . . '

THE EFFECTS OF INCREASING PRESSURE,
PADI OPEN WATER MANUAL, 1999–2007

By the time I return to London, I feel a little something like replenishment. It seems clearer to me with every dip under the water, with every splash of knowledge: the more I dive, the more I observe. The more I observe, the less I fear. And when it comes to the things I can't sit with yet, the things that instinctively make me fret, my plan is to prep myself until I can confront them – whether or not I happen to be near the sea.

If only I could dive into the underworld. Stick close to a trusted buddy, take a good look, then come up for air and hot chocolate. Instead, at my desk, during snatches of research time, I find a real-world way to keep progressing. When I first joined the PADI universe in Koh Tao, I hoped never to see the inside of a hyperbaric chamber. But now, I decide, that is going to change.

For fifteen years, London has been home to two hyper-baric chambers, one in the east, a bus ride from my new home, and one out in the west. Both are part-funded by the NHS, and offer free treatments to UK patients who need to be recompressed, as do all of the chambers belonging to the British Hyperbaric Association, based in locations that stretch from Plymouth to Orkney. Some of the chambers' users have contracted the bends while diving, and need to be put back at pressure in order to reabsorb the nitrogen bubbles that have been trapped in their blood or in tissues during ascent. Others enter a chamber not because of a diving incident, but because they have an ailment that can be treated by breathing in pure oxygen at pressure: diabetic ulcers, for instance; burns and radiotherapy damage too.

The west London chamber is where Vicky works – Vicky being the diver who almost got stuck at 100 metres, and who enthused about how exciting that high-risk depth was. It was she who told me about the 'dry dives' at her chamber, described on its website as 'the perfect environment to test a diver's ability at depth, but in a safe and water-free environ-ment . . . If a diver is underwater the first time they experience narcosis, they can panic and risk DCI [decompression illness; a.k.a. the bends]. A dry dive can prepare a diver mentally for what can happen underwater.'

I put in a request to 'dive' down to a pressure of 50 metres inside their chamber, 20 metres deeper than my body's ever experienced, and see how narcosis might affect me. As luck would have it, there's space for me to join a dry dive of 50 metres the following week. I claim it. In the meantime, I up the ante by contacting a diver who knows how to handle deep water more keenly than anyone else on the planet; a man Vicky herself has met, and describes as the most com-pelling diver imaginable. His name is Ahmed Gabr, and he has descended in scuba gear to an organ-crushing, world-beating depth of 332.35 metres; to the twilight zone and back – *without a sub.*

Vicky sends me his email address, stressing how useful anyone feeling fear would find it to talk to him, how he could probably keep me well on course to reaching the end of my project. Indeed, what she says about the methods surrounding deep-dive preparation feels just as relevant to my apprehension about one day meeting the whale shark, or even my own death, as the act of diving itself.

'No matter how much you prepare for it, you've never been there before,' she says. 'You don't know what it's going to be like . . . You can imagine it all you want, but it's your personal experience or how you feel on that day. It's a lot more in your head than anything physical. Everything else can be planned out to the tee, except your thoughts.'

Ahmed Gabr, more than most, must have a brilliant mastery over his mind. Clearly in awe, Vicky tells me, 'I've seen some of the footage of Ahmed sitting on the boat before he's on the world record dive and he's just looking at his watch a little bit, looking out to sea . . . You just think, *I do that before a dive.* Is it any different, my preparation, in actual reality, to his preparation? He's about to go and, like, *blow* his brains out to a depth that no one's ever been to. How the *eff* do you imagine that?'

I write to him and wait in hope of hearing the lessons he's learned. A massive, blank-eyed death-fish must be nothing to Ahmed Gabr.

During the countdown to my dry dive, one of Vicky's colleagues writes to say there's room for others to join me in the chamber – 'If you would like more company feel free to do some fast talking!' In an ideal world, Max would come along – getting narc'd together in a giant metal tube, what larks – but I discover it's not allowed. I've tried to convince him to learn some scuba, to be my long-term buddy, but Max still has no diving experience, and nor does he seem to want it. I've gone too far with the gruesome stories and anecdotes, sharing photos and videos that neither of us can unsee. Yuri Lipski. Shark attacks. The Byford Dolphin. At times I've even found myself in the weird position of trying to persuade him that scuba diving is perfectly safe and worthwhile. He can tell from the tone of my voice that it's a trap.

'You're going to be pressurised to 50 metres,' he repeats when I reveal my latest intentions. 'Couldn't that *give* you the bends?'

In an effort to deflect this troubling question, I ask if he'll extend the invite to his friends. There are three of them I know who like to dive, a chipper group of blokes who enjoy their adventures. The very next day their unanimous answer comes back. *No fucking way. Too dangerous.*

'It isn't,' I say to Max. 'Tell them it isn't. It can't be. These chambers are *NHS-approved*.'

Max raises his eyebrows. 'It sounds risky to me.'

The night before the dive I lie awake, thinking hard as usual. This time tomorrow I'll know what it's like to have entered both a hyperbaric chamber and a state of induced narcosis. I wonder if I'll also know what it's like to have the bends. Is this really something I want to be going through with?

When I first talked to Vicky about the topic of fear, she told me that 'the bravest thing when you're diving is to have the balls to call it'; to recognise your limits; cancel the dive as soon as it doesn't feel right, no matter what expectations others have of you. The problem is I don't know what's right and what isn't. If Max and his three friends think it's wrong, am I being an ignoramus by continuing?

I look at Max curled up beside me. His face is striped by moonlight passing through thin curtains that don't fully close. He's untroubled, asleep, breathing softly. I want to know how he does it.

The following morning, one part of my dilemma's decided for me. An emergency patient needs treating tonight, so my dry dive is being cancelled. I shock myself by feeling more disappointed than relieved. Without provocation I ask if I can rebook.

'Of course!' comes the reply. 'We're about to open a new set of dates. Keep checking back, and choose whichever you like.'

I check and check again and nothing happens. This looks like it might take a while, but I feel like I haven't got a while to wait. I write to the East London chamber, which is based at Whipps Cross Hospital. An amicable man named Wayne, the chamber's supervisor, gives me a call shortly afterwards. They do dry dives, he tells me, though only to 40 metres. He asks if I've got any friends I could pull together to make a dive group. ('Er . . . ' I fudge. 'Probably? Probably. I'd need to check, but probably.') Alternatively, Wayne suggests, if it's chambers and the bends I want to learn about, I could always come along for a little tour. I think for a second. Then: 'Thank you,' I say. 'You're on.'

What I expect before arriving at the chamber at London Hyperbaric Medicine (LHM) are dark, cramped rooms, stern people in lab coats and a potent smell of metal that sticks to the tongue. What I find when I turn up is nothing like that. Located inside a mobile building, on a quiet hospital side road, LHM is flooded with light, and festooned with hundreds of colourful 'Thank You' cards. Just a few feet away from reception, the hulking chamber hums and whirrs as if it is alive.

My friendly contact, Wayne, greets me by the desk, offers me tea, and leads me straight to a porthole on the side of the chamber itself.

'The patient said she doesn't mind you looking in,' he explains. 'She's having oxygen therapy to sort out a botched filler job on her lip.'

I peer through the circle of glass. The chamber seems large – big enough to fit eight divers at once. Wayne assures me; perfect for supporting large-scale crises like sat diving blowouts, where a whole team of divers like Bruce might need emergency treatment in one go. Inside it now sits a woman in green cotton scrubs. She's wearing a plastic hood over her head, and reading a magazine. Sure enough her lip looks sore, and Wayne tells me that a tube leading into the hood is currently pumping pure oxygen into her system.

'And there's Ronnie,' he says, pointing to a woman sitting opposite the patient; Ronnie being the head nurse. 'No one's ever in here on their own,' he adds.

I study a collection of fridge magnets stuck to the chamber's exterior – flashy trinkets gathered from across the world. Nearby, plastic shark toys lie on a ledge. The atmosphere in the room feels relaxed and harmless. Wayne's colleagues are happy to chat. While he fetches me a mug of tea, I ask the admin manager, Liz, if working at this chamber, seeing so many scuba casualties, has put her off going diving.

'Not at all,' she replies. 'Far from it.' Her answer seems sincere.

Wayne comes back not just with a tea for me, but also one for Ronnie. He leads me to the front of the chamber, and goes over the process of getting the tea inside: using a medical air lock and changing the pressure. A door is loosened, air whooshes out, tea goes in and comms are exchanged all the while. The door is closed, and within just a minute the lock is repressurised. Ronnie can grab her tea.

I learn that Wayne has worked at this chamber for twelve years; that he's an instructor too, as well as an ad hoc consultant for crews using diving in TV and movies. Wayne has seen all sorts of divers come through the doors, from those with the mildest symptoms (the majority that arrive here), to people who enter the chamber unable to move, and later are able to finish their treatment walking. As a result, there's little he doesn't know about the bends and how to get rid of it.

I start by asking Wayne if he's ever had decompression illness (DCI) himself after a dive. He nods and widens his eyes.

'I'm sure I've had it lots of times without really knowing,' he says. 'Years ago I instructed at all sorts of dive schools over in Thailand. Me and the other instructors had times where we were bouncing all day in the water, constantly going up and down, not giving ourselves enough time to decompress. Since I started working here I've realised that lots of things I dismissed as nothing were probably DCI. But people tell themselves it's something else: *my shoulders are probably sore from carrying air tanks; maybe I hit my elbow on the boat; I've got a headache because I didn't drink enough,* etc. The biggest problem with the bends is denial.'

I cannot help but think: *That's probably my biggest problem with most things.*

Wayne tells me that the majority of bends symptoms typically manifest between six and twelve hours after a dive. Patients who've become bent while still in the water are patients they see far less, since those are major emergency cases who need to be treated in chambers close to the dive site (usually nearer the coast). I then learn that DCI comes in two varieties. Physical bends – which present as pain only: a sore joint, for example; perhaps a rash – and neurological bends, which can involve numbness, tingling or headaches; even mood swings and memory loss. A UK diver who notices anything different about their body once they've ascended is advised to call the LHM hotline (open 24/7, 365 days a year), talk to one of the experts, and most probably head straight to their nearest chamber for further assessment. If it's needed, they may also begin their first recompression then. It's crucial, Wayne tells me, to seek out medical help as soon as possible, even when symptoms seem mild. If left for longer than seventy-two hours, the body starts reacting to nitrogen bubbles as if they're an infection. In defence it armours up, the soft, treatable bubbles become hard, and the process cannot be reversed. That's when cells can be damaged and destroyed.

Wayne tells me that so many divers he's met are nervous of getting in contact with the chamber, many because they believe that contracting the bends will show they're unskilled.

'Our busiest day should be Monday,' he says, given that most UK diving takes place at the weekend. 'But it's usually Wednesday or Thursday.' People leave it too long, he says. And when they do act, they waste their time heading to A&E, instead of contacting specialist hyperbaric staff straight away. As for the notion that being bent means you're not a good diver, Wayne assures me that skill has nothing to do with it. The fact is that anyone diving is at risk.

'There are only two ways to be guaranteed never to get the bends. Either you never go diving, or you dive and never come back up.'

I am trying to see this chamber, this nexus of so many fears, as a possible friend. It helps that Wayne refers to the machine as 'she' and 'her'. The idea of sitting inside it with a good book, soaking up pure oxygen, sounds not unlike a holiday.

And the fact that Brits get DCI treatment free in the UK, while other countries can charge $1000 per hour (or more) for the same service, well, it seems a waste *not* to be using it.

Triumphant, I put down my mug. 'I had thought going into the chamber would be risky,' I say, pleased to have been proved wrong. 'My boyfriend told me that if I did a dry dive I could end up getting bent.'

I chuckle at the thought. Then I notice that Wayne isn't joining in.

'It's *very* unlikely,' he says. 'But sometimes these things happen.'

My voice becomes small. 'Really?'

'Yeah,' says Wayne. 'That actually happened to me.' He tells me about an extreme day he once spent supervising patients. He became a little tired towards the end of it, was wearing a hood for staff members that required strong in-breaths to work, and probably wasn't inhaling his oxygen properly. When he finally got home and undressed for bed, his girlfriend spotted a purple rash over his ribs. It was a bend in his skin. Wayne came back as a patient the following day.

'But it's very rare,' he says. 'I was the third member of staff to be treated for DCI in the history of the chamber.' That's only three in over thirty years. And he says the rash went away fast.

There are other potential dangers in the chamber though, which I learn as Wayne warms to his theme. 'Ox-tox,' for example, or oxygen toxicity. This occurs when the patient's body absorbs *too much* oxygen during their treatment. As Wayne puts it, 'Humans are designed to breathe 21 per cent oxygen at surface, not 100 per cent oxygen at increased pressure.' Without breaks to take in normal air, internal body tissues can overload. The result is like an epileptic fit. Patients can knock themselves out cold, or end up unconsciously holding their breath, causing problems with lung expansion if the chamber's pressure lifts. There are also the risks that arise from wearing a plastic hood: potential asphyxiation should the air stop flowing through for any reason. ('What did your mother tell you never to do? Put a plastic bag over your head!') That's why this chamber always keeps a specialist sitting in with the patients, while another member of staff will externally monitor what's going on with CCTV.

The filler-job patient is almost at the end of her session, triggering a flurry of activity as the chamber winds down, bringing her and Ronnie back to 'surface'. The team here runs on checklists and protocol. Buttons are pressed, switches switched, messages transmitted through the speakers, and all is done with a well-rehearsed precision. As soon as the patient is out, reunited with her waiting dad and partner, Wayne beckons me to the open chamber entrance.

'Here we go,' he says. 'Have a look in.'

In my mind, I transform the chamber into a fish. A giant one at that. Taking a breath, I walk up the ramp and pass through the hefty door that would be her mouth. Her interior is like a small submarine, or the inside of a military aircraft. It's functional, largely metal, and lined with equipment. At the back, her tail end, is a smaller chamber room with another external entrance. Patients can use this room to go to the toilet during their treatment if needed, Wayne explains. Or, if multiple patients are in, and one needs to come out, that person can be ushered this way and their pressure altered separately from the main chamber.

They seem to have thought of everything.

What I had not thought of, what I'd not even considered, in spite of my chat with bathynaut Jon Copley, is perhaps the biggest danger of being sealed inside a hyperbaric chamber: the risk of fire. With pure oxygen on tap, and nowhere to run, a flame or flash of static in this chamber mid-treatment could be disastrous – a bigger catastrophe here than in a deep-sea sub, for sure, thanks to the nearby abundance of oxygen cylinders. Wayne shows me a list of no-nos that is taped to a standing post by the chamber door. Everything on it is banned. Among the more obvious candidates – the mobile phones, lighters and lithium batteries – is a selection of more surprising potential combustibles. Perfume, sugar, talc, make-up, fountain pens. Newspapers too, are out of bounds. The print itself is flammable, while the paper itself is far too effective a kindling. Even grease is off limits.

'No cream cakes then,' I say. 'No oily takeaways.'

'Definitely not,' says Wayne.

'Salmon?'

'Salmon's all right. Unless you add mayo.'

Nurse Ronnie overhears our conversation. She says if I want to know even more, I could come to a special training day they're running. It would be my chance to see their fire prevention system at work. So it is that, not long afterwards, I'm back at the chamber again, wondering how knowledge can be so scary, when according to Rob from Help for Heroes, it's supposed to make my fears go away.

At the training day, I meet various staff who work at the hospital chamber, principally doctors and nurses. We sit in rows in a small grey room as Steve, a hyperbaric supervisor and ex-police diver, goes through a PowerPoint presentation on hyperbaric fires. He tells us that one chamber a year worldwide is destroyed by fire. A few gasps of disbelief pass through the room. More audible shock arises when he goes into some of the details. In Florida in 2012, for example, during an oxygen treatment for cerebral palsy, a small boy and his grandmother died when the boy brought out his toy car – one that was set in motion by pulling its tyres back against the ground. The spark from that moment of friction ignited the chamber, where the flames burned for five minutes before the door could even be opened. Fifteen years before that, in Milan, eleven people died when a man carried a charcoal handwarmer into his treatment. Though the fire was extinguished quickly, it consumed all the chamber's oxygen in just thirty seconds. Those who had survived the flames were rapidly killed by asphyxiation instead.

Steve then plays us a video. It is made by a German company which manufactures fire systems for chambers, and demonstrates, in a series of unflinching lab clips, the speed at which small increases in pressure and oxygen can massively accelerate the ferocity of flames. Most terrifying of all is a fire test involving a dummy dressed in a non-cotton, synthetic shirt. As soon as the flame catches on to it, heat flashes across the fabric like lightning, transforming it into a hard shell that nothing can penetrate – not water, nor even further flames. As a result, the fire continues to burn underneath it, long after the sprinkler system has gone off. No water can get through to put it out. The flames can't dance free to be dowsed.

'If fire could dream,' says the video, 'it would dream for a hyperbaric chamber.'

I sit in my chair fully rigid, vowing to clear out all my synthetic garments when I get home.

'That,' says Wayne, turning to face us from the front row, 'is why *only* 100 per cent cotton scrubs are allowed inside our chamber.'

I make a note: *MUST check pants*.

Next it's time to test the chamber's sprinkler system. I volunteer to be among the few who are inside it when the sprinklers go off, and change into a set of cotton scrubs with the rest of our skittish group.

'It's going to be freezing,' we're warned. 'The chamber is

programmed to virtually flood when the fire alarm goes off. Are you sure you want to do this?'

In the spirit of using knowledge to my advantage, I speak up. 'I'm sure.' If I'm ever in a chamber with a fire, it'd be nice to remember how that fire could be put out. But as we go in, I'm having second thoughts. I'm not the only one.

'I'm scared,' says one of the doctors.

'Me too,' says admin manager Liz. 'The waiting is the worst bit.'

'Remind me again why I'm in here?' asks a nurse, in a voice that tries, but fails, to sound like a joke.

Liz is right. The waiting is unpleasant. There's a leaden tension in the air and, as the heavy door seals us in, that tension thickens. We look at each other, anticipating an imminent rush of cold water. We've been told it'll be so strong we won't be able to see in front of us. That it'll go on for several minutes before we can leave.

There's a knock on the window: Wayne. It's the signal for one of us 'patients' to shout fire. After that there'll be a brief pause, and the floods will come. I giggle loosely, all nerves. Liz winces. Bracing herself, she shouts out 'Fire!'

The five of us stiffen up. 'Oh God,' the nurse is saying. 'Oh God, oh God.' I feel very much like we're hanging off a precipice, about to plunge 100 metres down.

A moment later I'm yelping involuntarily as strong jets of water blast from pipes above us. As promised, the water is cold. So cold that I am shivering. But it's also a relief to know I'm no longer on fire. As I clutch my arms and jog on the spot to stay warm, artificial rain pastes my scrubs against me, and I realise that this could be a handy lesson in anticipation: of how the build-up can so often be worse than the main event.

Maybe that means it's best not to wait. To avoid anticipation at all costs. Maybe when it comes to new things I should just fucking do it, swimming with the whale shark first and foremost. Until I hear back from Ahmed Gabr, an expert in patience and prep, and am forced to consider that, in certain situations, just fucking doing it might risk fucking things up.

In 2014, with a support team of around thirty crew in tow (medics, divers and the like), Ahmed Gabr, an ex-special forces officer from the Egyptian army, and an experienced technical diver, embarked on a pioneering expedition to become the deepest diver ever. He was keen to discover how far one person could go – 'there was no research established' – and aimed to plunge 350 metres beneath the water off Dahab to find out. (Coincidentally the spot was not too far from the Blue Hole, the dive site which claimed the life of Yuri Lipski.) In the event, hampered by the onset of some serious physical issues, Ahmed officially made it to just over 332 metres before turning around.

At 332 metres, water pressure is more than thirty-three times greater than it is at the surface. At 332 metres, the sea is officially twilight, also known as the mesopelagic, where only 1 per cent of surface light shines through. In certain parts of the world, this zone is also the realm of the giant spider crab, a spindly crustacean measuring almost 4 metres across. It is a daytime home for lanternfish, a species named for its powers of luminescence, and a battleground for Harryhausen-style tussles between sperm whales and giant squid. In other words, the realm is a realm of the epic.

It's appropriate, then, that Ahmed Gabr, in returning from that, is a legend; nothing less than a diving superstar. More people have walked on the moon (twelve) than have done what Ahmed alone has achieved. Yet, speaking from an office out in Cairo, sharing his tips about unknowns and fears with me on a Saturday morning, he tells me he needed a long time to work out whether or not to go ahead with his plan.

'There was a big question,' he says. 'It took me first two years to assess myself: can I actually do it, or do I just *think* I can do it? It's a huge difference between who you are and who you think you are.' Ahmed says he had to be sure his motives for completing the dive were pure. That he wasn't taking it on to boost his ego. That his desire to go deep wouldn't cloud his judgment or threaten his safety during the dive itself.

He explains how he started to hide his plans from certain people near him, otherwise 'they got amazed with what I'm doing. They liked it very much; they started to create a kind of a peer pressure around me ... The moment I start to feel like I'm very full of myself, I have to put my foot on the floor.'

Ahmed enlisted the help of a mentor, who, after unsuccessfully trying to change his mind, then helped him slowly train towards his goal. As part of their preparation, Ahmed tells me, he dived 'to the maximum of the earth crack itself, in the south of Egypt' – a phenomenal 209 metres. He made it a priority to experiment with his own capabilities, pushing his boundaries further every time. But even then he was not sure he was ready, and Ahmed knew that to go without being ready had a high risk of costing his life. 'I delayed my record actually five times.' When word got out about what he was doing, 'I heard a lot of things,' says Ahmed. 'I heard myself described like I'm an attention seeker, a deceiver, trying to extort to expand my business. I heard it said that I'm depressed; I'm trying to commit suicide.' In response he created a psychological bubble around him. Nothing was allowed to penetrate it. Within this bubble he focused on 'visualisation, anticipation, and then breathing – every slight change in my breathing at that depth, it might lead to a disaster afterward. I have to be mentally completely stable. I have to keep my track.'

Ahmed tells me he was afraid, but did not give his fear the space to control him. Every morning he trained physically, as he was used to doing in the army. Every day he prepared scenarios, largely hypothetical. He tried to plan to mitigate the risks. With the help of his team, he calculated every aspect of the dive as best he could: the tanks, the timings, nutrition, decompression. But one risk could not be planned for: the effect of the depth itself.

'There's no risk mitigation with that,' says Ahmed, speaking as if he's reliving that time again. 'That's why I'm there: to explore *exactly* how I am going to be there, how my body's going to react.'

On a September morning, in view of a Guinness World Records adjudicator, following six years of self-assessment, risk preparation, team building and postponements, Ahmed entered the water and began to follow his long guide rope down. His speed was quick. It had to be. Ahmed knew that if he didn't start heading back up within fifteen minutes, he would not have enough air to reach his first support diver on the ascent.

But first, at 290 metres' depth, still making his descent, Ahmed started to feel the effects of high-pressure nervous syndrome (HPNS) – a syndrome that causes tremors, nausea and dizziness; all major threats to his performance, and chances of survival. Eight metres deeper his dive computers stopped working, removing his personal references to the depth. Ahmed stayed with the rope, which was marked with measuring tags, and continued to go down, wondering whether to call the dive, or whether he could safely endure both HPNS and the 'big hallucination factor'.

I listen, enthralled, scribbling notes to help me. *Motives pure? Worth it?? NEED TEAM. Mitigate. ARGH.* My phobia quest looks like child's play in comparison.

I ask Ahmed what he saw down there. If he was able to see anything. Big fish, maybe. Sharks. Worse. Despite the internal struggle he went through, he explains how part of him witnessed the totally inhuman world around him.

'Colours changed back then,' he recalls. 'I saw twilight for the first time in my life, and then complete darkness down there.' Approximately twelve minutes after leaving the surface, he reached the deepest point he would get to, collecting a tag that marked it as 335 metres (a result later adjusted to 332.5 because of an alleged kink in the rope). It would take Ahmed far, far longer to safely get back up to the human world. Meanwhile, still at depth, the tremors were making him lose control of his extremities – he was not able to regain them until he ascended a further 75 metres. At the same time, other effects were compromising his safety. The depth was making him mentally confused. He was coughing into his regulator. He had contracted pulmonary oedema: fluid on the lungs that can lead to respiratory failure. Knowing that neither rushing nor taking a break were options for him, Ahmed kept heading up slowly, carefully, using all his energy to stay calm and maintain focus. Fear was not allowed to enter his bubble.

Bubble, I write, underlining it, *equals NO FEAR.*

I need bubble.

At 110 metres, Ahmed reached the first of many support divers, a meticulous relay of team mates each dipping down to play their part in the drama. Accompanied the rest of the way, gently rising in stages for many hours to offset even the smallest chance of the bends, Ahmed finally breached the Red Sea's surface to a hero's welcome, 13 hours and 50 minutes after ending his descent.

Though initially able to stand and talk to the crowd, the effects of his dive were to dog Ahmed for some time.

'A few hours afterwards I wasn't a hundred per cent OK,' he says. 'I could feel it, my metabolism, the way I feel, the way I talk even, my desire – I felt something different. The chemistry of my body completely changed, you know?' Ahmed had a bend in his skin, for starters. He was also dehydrated – and stayed that way for two months. The effects of the pulmonary oedema lasted for two whole years. But all the problems went away eventually, he says. 'I'm recovered completely right now.'

I ask Ahmed if he ever thought about dying, whether during the prep for his attempt, throughout the course of the record dive itself, or while adjusting to his subsequent altered state. Death must have been so close to him at times, waiting in the blackness, hoping he might spend a few minutes more, coaxing him to the very end of the rope. As I wait for his answer I see the big fish lurking in the shadows, a large mouth twitching in time with Ahmed's tremors – the shark that summoned him down there, willing him to test himself against it. But if Ahmed sees the beast too he doesn't say. He shrugs it off.

'If it's your day it's your day,' he says. Then he smiles into the webcam, delivering a line he must have spoken many times before. 'I believe everyone dies. But not everyone can live.'

13

Woman Alive

I want to live a life of discovery. I want a life where I finish what I start. I want to swim with the world's biggest fish and survive.

I want to keep going.

I want to be better.

Methodical and controlled, like Ahmed in the twilight – applying his brain to the task, to logistics, not the crushing excess of sea over his head – I gather all the anecdotes I have about swimming with the whale shark. From Sam, the woman I interviewed at James Deane's shop, who snorkelled with a whale shark in the Maldives. From a young guy called Chris, who once saw four whale sharks on a single diving holiday, and almost collided with one of them. From Vas, the mine diver built like Action Man, who said that he was startled by one in a sudden submerged encounter.

I hear the experience described as 'alienating' and 'nerve-wracking'.

'Incredible,' says one woman.

'Totally prehistoric,' says another.

Every morning I contact dive shops around the world. Look up prices for flights and hotels. Consider suggestions like Honduras, the Seychelles, Galapagos, the Azores – even a tuna-processing plant off the coast of New Jersey. No one I talk to will promise a sighting, however. It seems nobody can.

Undeterred, I pick over screens filled with pictures. I read as many articles as I can find. In one of them, an expert explains that, of all the whale shark categories, juvenile female whale sharks – the ones that have survived a dangerous youth and are close to being ready to have their own pups – are the most important part of the population in terms of conservation. Without safeguarding these females first and foremost, the species will die out. But these females are also the part of the population we know the least about.

Juvenile males usually stay near the coast, says the expert. But aside from a few coastal stragglers, nobody knows where the juvenile females are going. Or why they separate from the males for so long.

Nobody knows if these females are OK.

As I'm trawling through the internet, trying to work out the shape of my fate more clearly, I return again and again to Wildbook for Whale Sharks, the global 'visual database of ... encounters and of individually catalogued whale sharks.' Anyone who sees a whale shark can take a photograph of the animal's left flank, and Wildbook will let them know if the shark has been sighted before – and who it is. Perhaps it will be Stella. A-670. Sharkira. Or perhaps they've come fin to fin with the mighty Buttermouth. (Could I really be afraid of a fish if I knew its name was Buttermouth?)

I discover that Wildbook has logged over fifty thousand whale shark sightings since the project began in the early noughties, identifying each one of them using NASA technology: mapping their markings like constellations. According to the stats, just under six thousand 'citizen scientists' have contributed to their overall findings so far. (Though there's no metric to tell how panicked these citizens were while snapping their photos.)

I take a punt and write to the guy who set the whole thing up. His name is Jason Holmberg and he lives in Portland, Oregon. I want to know if he's ever been scared of whale sharks; if he'll talk to me about his own encounters; if he'll admit to filling his trunks within the presence of a monster. He responds to my email with the pleasing speed you'd expect from someone whose career revolves around software, and we soon have a date to Skype.

'Interacting with a small whale shark versus interacting with a massive whale shark is a very different experience,' Jason tells me. It's a Friday morning in Oregon, and the noise of his kids occasionally makes its way through to our call. It sounds like they're having a great time, and no wonder: their dad has swum with more than ten whale sharks and lived. These children are the offspring of a leading light in modern conservation, a man who has helped put software in place to monitor numerous threatened species, including seals, manta rays, sperm whales and polar bears.

'Small whale sharks, I feel, there's a certain amount of understanding you can build with the animal,' Jason continues. 'And I think it's a matter of scale ... The first whale shark I was in the water with was 8 foot, in Djibouti. It was very curious about me, I was very curious about it. There was a fair amount of contact time just looking at each other, exploring each other.'

An 8-foot long whale shark is 2 feet longer than I am. Instinctively I look up at the ceiling of my bedroom. If that whale shark was here it would fill this place. I imagine something that large exploring me now. It's impossibly creepy.

Jason, meanwhile, has moved on to higher things.

'When I was in the water with a 40-foot pregnant female off the Galapagos, I was in the water with a leviathan,' he says. 'I just didn't register. That animal has moved to a psychological place that is beyond me, you know what I mean?'

'Yes,' I say, with feeling. 'I think I do.'

'I didn't—' Jason stops himself. 'How do I explain it? I feel like I was in *its* world, you know?'

He tells me about the time he swam with a giant manta ray for half an hour, the pair of them keeping at touching distance all the while; that he once sat with his arm around a beluga whale – that together they watched the dolphins swim past, like a couple of lovers gazing out to sea on a tropical honeymoon.

'A whale shark at 40 foot is different,' he says. 'That sense of empathy and connection isn't there. Just the opposite. It's like watching a giant walk by.' Forty foot is one-and-a-half times the length of a classic London bus. Two adult giraffes stacked one on top of the other. It sounds too big to be real for just one animal. A single, non-empathetic, drifting shark. I cannot imagine that meeting. I ask him how he felt.

'Like I was invading,' Jason says.

My skin bristles. I am picturing what those powerful fish might do in response to a threat. How could anyone stay in place with a creature that large fee-fi-foh-fumming in close proximity? I ask if the sensation made Jason want to rocket out of the water, as I fear it would for me.

'No,' he says. 'It just made me feel like I certainly wasn't a part of something grander.'

For a moment that comment gets stuck in my eardrums.

Then the sense of the words filters through. *Not part of something grander.* As soon as the meaning hits me, I feel winded. This is not what I'd expected from someone who'd swum with a full-sized whale shark. This is not what I hoped I would hear. Too often this year, I've felt like I'm not part of something grander; as if, in the end, loss and disappointment could be all there is. And that's not a feeling I want to feel any more strongly.

I remark on how isolating his interpretation sounds. Jason agrees. But he does not talk like a man who has been plunged into a crisis of existence.

'It makes me understand how much of this animal's life history is simply beyond me,' he explains. Jason tells me that no one has ever been able to map the migration routes of a large, pregnant female whale shark. No one has ever seen mating. No one has ever seen birth. Not *one* researcher has been able to track a whale shark for as long as a single year.

'So this is an animal that's spending all of its life far away from me, at depths that my body couldn't handle, going through a life history we don't understand, that we can't observe. If this thing was literally travelling to the bottom of the ocean through a wormhole to another planet and then coming back every year – well, no one can say it's not, right?'

That evening, over a pasta dinner, Max asks how my call with Jason went. I tell him I don't quite know. Then I correct myself.

'Pretty well, I think.'

'What did you learn that was useful?'

'Lots. But mostly that I need to know much more.'

'That's exciting,' says Max. He swallows a forkful of food and looks at me. Clears his throat. 'Is something wrong?'

I ponder this for a moment, staring down at my plate of food. Tentacles of spaghetti coil beneath an olive oil slick. Gradually I realise I am knocking my knife handle against the table. *Tic-tic-tic-tic-tic-tic-tic-tic.*

'Are you thinking about Granny?' asks Max.

Tic-tic-tic-tic-tic.

Max reaches out. Takes the knife off me.

'What if, when I find the whale shark, it's a let-down? What if I'm still afraid?'

Max shrugs. 'Then at least you'll know.'

The more I learn about whale sharks, the more elusive they get. I speak to the director of the world's only Whale Shark and Oceanic Research Centre, based on the island of Utila in Honduras. He tells me that peak whale shark season there usually involves around twenty-five sightings in two months, but during the last peak season, the number of sightings was only four.

'Something's going on,' he says, 'something's changing; we just don't know what it is.'

I ask him where I should go if I want to see them. He suggests checking out Mozambique, where a well-respected NGO conducts research on marine megafauna. It'd be worth contacting them too, he says. I add the NGO to my list – *Marine Megafauna Foundation: CONTACT* – only so I can tick them off as soon as I send them a message, five minutes later.

Next I get hold of a dive instructor in Mozambique. She has seen hundreds in the water there and recommends a visit. Except there's a caveat.

'It's not like a congregation of whale sharks,' she says over Skype. 'It's more like a passing through as they're feeding, so we will get, you know, two or three over the course of a week on average.' Which means that in certain weeks they find none at all. 'Whenever there's no plankton they go to the depths. They can do that for up to two or three months before they get too cold.'

I can't afford to stay out in Mozambique for up to three months just waiting, so I continue the search, venturing up every avenue I find. It is then that I come across Georgia Aquarium. Located in Atlanta, America – not the Georgia bordering Russia and Azerbaijan – from 2005 to 2012 it was the largest aquarium in the world. (Today that title belongs to a Chinese attraction.) One of Georgia Aquarium's main draws is its Ocean Voyager exhibit, a 6.3-million-gallon tank containing 425 square metres of viewing windows, thousands of fish, four manta rays and . . . four whale sharks.

'Georgia Aquarium is the only location in the world where diving face-to-fin with whale sharks, the largest fish on earth, is guaranteed,' says its website. Which, potentially, makes it the only way I'll meet the giant fish I've been seeking. But the idea of spotting a whale shark in a tank seems far too much like cheating – *Moby-Dick* ending with Ahab finding the white whale through the phone book. If my whale shark can't hide or disappear, if it is not the master, or mistress, of its own space, I wonder what it would actually represent. A hollow victory, maybe.

I am confused. And conflicted. Reading more web pages doesn't help. The aquarium seems to pride itself on its status as a place to educate visitors on the state of our seas and their inhabitants. At the same time, when I look up the aquarium's whale shark history online, it isn't long before I find national news reports of two whale sharks that died in their care. I consider the possibility that my own desires, and the desires of others like me – people who, for whatever reason, want the experience of these leviathans up close – have created an extreme artificial environment in which the health of an officially 'vulnerable' species comes second to the wishlists of homo sapiens.

I would like to find out more, so write to the aquarium enquiring about the possibility of a chat. A chirpy woman in their comms department responds within a few days, and requests all my questions by email. I send them over.

While I wait to hear the results, Simon Pierce, co-founder of the Marine Megafauna Foundation, writes back to me; a big contact for big fish. Simon says he will be in London soon after completing a project in Svalbard. We may be able to meet up and talk about fear and whale sharks then. He can even give me some travelling tips.

My plates are starting to spin again. I feel like I'm regaining focus. More so when a document of answers arrives from the aquarium. I tuck in, eager to learn. I discover that Georgia Aquarium has had whale sharks in its possession since 2006, when two females were transported there from Taiwan. One year later, two male whale sharks followed. They were all acquired from legal Taiwanese fisheries, I'm told, and were therefore saved from being sold into the fish market. Whether the sharks were caught specifically to be sold to the Georgia Aquarium is not made clear, but one line states that they were brought to Atlanta to 'serve as ambassadors for their species', making it sound like something the whale sharks signed up for – or would have done, if only they'd had the opposable joints required to write their consent. Whatever, it seems their services to the species are non-retractable.

'We have made a commitment to care for these animals for the entirety of their lives,' the document says. 'Additionally, it would be next to impossible to transport them safely back to Taiwan, where they would have to be released, and it would be very difficult to obtain the proper permitting.'

I also learn about how these sharks reached America: each was placed in a specially designed life-support container inside a cargo aircraft, and taken on a thirty-hour, monitored journey. Why did they make that journey? Because the founder of the aquarium had a dream: 'to bring the ocean to Atlanta ... [giving] millions of guests the opportunity to see a species they most likely would never have a chance to see'. Atlanta, it should be noted, is 267 miles from its nearest stretch of coastline.

When I reach the end of this document, I notice that a few key questions I asked about the whale sharks have not been answered. Though I did write that, if the respondents were tight on time, they should prioritise the questions that they thought most important, it's interesting to see exactly which were omitted. Which were deemed to be not important enough.

Of my original nineteen questions, only four have been left out:

- Do you think that being in captivity impacts on the whale sharks' mental or physical health?
- Do the sharks ever try to dive deep in the tank? I understand this is something they do in open ocean.
- What do you think the main positives are about having whale sharks in captivity? On the flip-side, what are the negatives?
- I understand that whale sharks have died at the aquarium in the past. Would you be able to tell me the details?

When I enquire as to why these statements went unanswered, I'm advised that the one about death was ignored inadvertently. As for the rest of them, the aquarium team 'provided responses that were the most applicable and relevant

to [my] project.' For a minute I'm thrown by the comment –
how can they know my project so well, when *I'm* not always
sure what I'm doing? – but I keep the confusion to myself
and download the latest attachment.

In this updated document, aquarium staff expand about
the losses of whale sharks Norton and Ralph in 2007, which
were probably, they speculate, due to a treatment delivered
'to remove a parasite from the system'. Animal autopsies were
performed, with tissues and other structures used in scientific
research for 'a better understanding of whale shark feeding mechanisms and the eventual sequencing of the whale
shark genome.'

Further information about the dark side notwithstanding,
the rest of the knowledge that the staff at Georgia Aquarium
do impart helps build a clearer picture of what to expect when
humans dive with whale sharks – or captive whale sharks, at
least. I learn that the sharks are constantly swimming, unless
feeding vertically in the water; that, on the whole, they seem
indifferent to interactions with people – that only sometimes
do they seem curious. Immediately my fear-brain decides that
I would be one of those 'sometimes' people, a diver the sharks
would not only notice, but relentlessly hone in on. I'm told,
however, that the vast majority of aquarium visitors who see
the whale sharks there react with joy and awe rather than fear,
let alone Jason Holmberg's sense of isolation.

'Most of our guests have never seen a whale shark in person
before,' says the document. '[S]ome have never been to the
ocean at all.' Occasionally, yes, some panic while in the tank.
But when this happens staff employ a technique that seems
to calm most of them down: 'with the assistance of the Dive
Immersion Program staff and taking some time to calmly
float on the surface, they eventually relax and recognize the
animals are not interested in them at all.'

This seems like the kind of approach that CBT gurus would applaud – and exactly the sort of thing I might need to try if I find myself in a similar position. Only, I'm now even less convinced that Georgia Aquarium is where I want to go. On the plus side, the organisation is a not-for-profit venture, with its own respected research and conservation team. But – and it seems like a massive *but* – there's the fact that, so far, six wild whale sharks have been caught in Taiwan, flown to America, and encased in a single tank so that passing humans can gawp at something new.

I hope Simon Pierce, the megafauna man, can offer me an alternative when we meet. If not, I am stumped. With no one else able to promise me a sighting of a whale shark, no one guaranteeing my trip will be worth it, this trail could go cold.

I wonder if I could ever let go of the whale shark. I wonder if any old big fish would do. While it's true that finding the whale shark has now been my only constant for two years, I can't shake the feeling that the Number One Swimming Tarantula might actually be a red herring. Perhaps there's an easier way to conquer this fear – and help me move towards addressing the others.

Killing time on a train ride to visit my mum, I latch on to the carriage's pokey wifi and investigate alternative big fish. In moments, I learn that the world's *second* biggest fish is the basking shark. The basking shark is harmless and can be dived with in the UK.

Still curious, I dig deeper.

In the Isle of Man and in Cornwall, the viewing figures for basking sharks convey that all-too-familiar unpredictability. Hit and miss. Then I find a website boasting 100 per cent success rates for its previous year of basking shark encounters in the Hebrides. One hundred per cent is my favourite rate when it comes to success. Disbelieving but intrigued, I give them a call. My phone won't connect. Bloody train.

I try again while walking from the station towards Mum's house. This time I get through.

'That's right,' says a man named Shane, the company's owner. 'All our four-day tours last year saw basking sharks.'

I can't believe what I'm hearing. Could this actually be a *predictable* giant shark – one that's not even inside an aquarium?

I ask him how big they are.

'We sometimes get individuals that are over 10 metres long up here.'

'Ten metres?'

'Or bigger.'

Ten metres is more than ten paces. I count the distance walking between the lampposts on Bournemouth Road. It takes me nearly ten seconds to walk the whole length of one fish. If this man is telling the truth, if these 10-metre-plus sharks really exist, they are larger than the juvenile whale sharks in Georgia.

My fingers start to tingle.

'Do you know where these basking sharks are, then?' I ask.

'We sure do,' Shane replies. 'A big group of them stay off the island of Coll. There's about twenty-five of them in a bay near here right now. The weather's perfect at the moment too – flat-calm and sunny – so if you came up here tomorrow, say, you'd be just about guaranteed a swim with them.'

'Not a dive?'

'No. Snorkelling's the best way with these guys.'

My heart is audibly thumping. This is all so sudden and unexpected. I pause by an overgrown hedge to make calculations. Coll is about 600 miles away from where I am standing. If I hired a car it would take me at least thirteen hours to make the journey. I look at my watch. It's after 9 p.m. The car rental shops around here will be closed already. Besides, Mum is waiting for me right now, possibly in her dressing gown. If I can make my way up to Scotland at a later date though, if the basking sharks appear, if I can cope with one of those and keep going, then maybe, just maybe, I'll be cured. And if I'm not? Then I'll still have the option of finding the world's biggest fish.

'I won't be able to get to Coll tomorrow,' I say. 'But I prob-ably could do a four-day tour with more notice.'

'Great,' says Shane, 'we'd love to have you. Just one thing that's worth mentioning: we were lucky last year – we had at least one day on each four-day tour, weather-wise, that let us get out to where we needed to go. We know that the basking sharks *will* be there. But if the weather gets bad and stays bad, there's a small possibility we might not be physically able to travel across to them. We'll still have a good time and take you to other places, but you *might* not get a chance to swim with the sharks. It's *very* unlikely. But possible.'

The next morning, before breakfast, overlooked by a framed passport photo of Granny Codd, I transfer the money to Shane.

14

Open-Mouthed

'*What you don't know* can *hurt you.*'

HOW TO USE THIS MANUAL AND SUCCEED IN THE
COURSE, PADI OPEN WATER MANUAL, 1999–2007

My mother's best friend from college had a brother who wrote a book. His name was Alex Wright, and his book was called *The Dream of Hieronymus Sloth*. Eventually it was published by his father. In part of this book, the author portrayed a disturbing, dream like event. He wrote about a macabre scene of death; of seeing a limb detached on damp ground, a group huddled around it in 'mortal terror'.

Last night I could barely sleep, so I'm out of bed early, wondering how to calm down, when I notice the book on my mother's lounge shelves. At once I recall the postscript: that *Hieronymus Sloth* was published posthumously; that Alex, the author, was involved in a motorbike accident that killed him. One uncanny feature of the crash was that it severed his right arm. Another was that the night when it happened was misty. Damp. The details he had written down – the detached limb, the wet ground, the mortal terror – had fatally come to pass.

I think of the possibility that, if I meet a basking shark, my story might suddenly end in one of the nightmarish ways I've imagined. By the time anyone reads about it, I'll have been retrieved, face down, from the Scottish sea. Or the current will have carried me away. Perhaps both things will happen, and I'll have inhaled the third of a can of water it takes for a human to drown.

Stop. Breathe. Relax.

Searching for more stabilising thoughts, I remember something Mungo mentioned, when we sat in the pub in London. He told me about a frenzy of creatures he dived with during a sardine run in South Africa. I wanted to know how he composed himself among feeding bull sharks, copper sharks, dusky sharks, whales and dolphins. All of them were significantly bigger and faster than he could ever be. All of them were speeding past him, jaws springing, to reach either the sardines, or the sardine-eaters. And Mungo said, 'These sharks are incredible and graceful. Actually, you know what, it sounds stupid but if one was to take me, it would be an amazing death. And I probably wouldn't feel much because they're so effective at killing, it'd be like, you know, *it's over* . . .

'I think you'd zone out,' he continued. 'I don't think there'd be too much pain. The times when I've really injured myself, when I've seen bones sticking out of me, I've been all right. I've thought, *I actually feel quite superhuman right now.*'

I try to think more like Mungo. To use the adrenaline as my anaesthetic. If things do end up going wrong in Scotland, could thirty minutes surrounded by sharks be a greater way to experience life than thirty years sedately spent at home?

After talking to Shane and sending him money, after pelting my mother with questions and being warned to change the subject ('I don't *know* if you've made the right decision,

Georgina. It's not for me to say'), I start to secretly test myself with photographs of basking sharks. In terms of fearsome appearances, this creature has an edge on most of its cousins. Forget even the great white shark with its shocking red gums and dagger-teeth. A basking shark's mouth, I've decided, speaks death in volumes. It's a vortex of horror. A gaping chasm lined with skeletal strips. Even though I know the species (probably) does not work for the Grim Reaper. Even though, like the whale shark, they are (in theory) harmless.

It takes a great deal of effort to try and desensitise myself to the sight of a shark silently screaming through the water. Sometimes staring at images makes me calmer. Sometimes it does not. Often, no matter the number of blogs that tell me they're only gaping along to eat plankton, the knowledge simply refuses to settle my nerves. The gap between words and feelings is oil and water; no dilution.

While great whites could be classed as the chainsaw-wielding menaces of nightmares – brash and quick, but ultimately conquerable – basking sharks could be better than even whale sharks at playing the spectre. The fact that this spectre might not touch you isn't the point. If it appears by your bed you know, you *know*, you're finished.

'I think you might be overthinking it,' says Mum, when I once again voice my concerns, this time while she's trying to send an email. 'Nobody knows what's around the corner, so drop it for now and do something else.' She points at the dog who is glaring at me, a tennis ball in his mouth. 'Like taking him to the park. And finally throwing that ball for him.'

I take her advice. Walk the dog. Throw the ball. Try to let go of my thoughts and focus on what's around me. (This grass. That tree branch. My clenched, white fist.) Doing that works up to a point, but back in London I have more night-mares, despite the fact I'm meditating more than ever; despite all the times I've dived with fish and come back safely to land. Never mind that basking sharks aren't even the biggest sharks out there.

My subconscious has gone into overdrive. One night I have a terrible dream about being in the water with a sperm whale. It is hooked by a line, blood pours from its mouth, and it is looking right at me. I am so repelled by the sight I cannot save it. After ages trying to escape, I force myself awake in a hot sweat of shame.

Max slurs, 'Whasthmatter.'

'Sperm whales,' I whisper.

'Mm.'

In my waking hours, time speeds up. Almost out of nowhere, it seems, and just a few weeks pre-Scotland, Simon Pierce arrives in town, representing the Marine Megafauna Foundation. The world's biggest fish is on the agenda again. It will not be contained. With the subject of whale sharks resurfacing, I'm reminded of how formidable, how frighteningly irresistible, this species of fish has been to me for so long.

I feel like I should cling to Simon like a lifebuoy or lucky charm. This is someone who knows whale sharks better than most. And he also knows where to find them.

'I'm in an incredibly privileged position,' he confides soon after we meet, 'to be able to see whale sharks in the wild pretty much whenever I feel like ...

'But I do try to be modest,' he adds. 'Or at least appear so.'

It was Simon who co-wrote the whale shark's IUCN listing, compiling all the official stats I've read about its habits and numbers, helping to reclass the species as 'Endangered'. I want to ply him with drinks and food for his time, so we meet at Borough Market – he in his shorts and sunglasses, the marine biologist's uniform – and head for the nearest selection of good cakes. After ordering two large slices, and talking in depth about pavlovas (a dessert claimed by New Zealand, Simon's home country, as its own), we move on to a topic I can't bring myself to abandon: what really is known right now about the largest fish on our planet? And could one ever swallow me whole?

Simon animatedly starts by addressing my second question. 'Whale sharks are actually very aware of what's going through their mouth,' he says. 'I've seen them ingest jellyfish by accident, and they kind of, *puh*—' He mimes spitting something out.

I tell him the story I heard about a man swimming into a whale shark's mouth, killing both himself and the shark.

Simon rolls his eyes. 'Never happened.'

'Oh.'

I ask him about the YouTube video where the whale shark keeps pushing and pushing at the divers. Surely that's clear evidence that these sharks can take issue with humans. Simon knows the video I mean, and voices a strong suspicion that those sharks were from an area where they were used to being hand-fed.

'They're not aggressive,' he tells me. 'They would just like food. Some of them are interested in bubbles from air tanks too.'

After more fear-based probing of this variety, more by-products of my nerves, Simon reveals that there is only one whale shark individual he knows of that doesn't seem to like being around people – but that, instead of reacting viciously, she only ever chooses to swim away.

'I think of whale sharks as being ocean Labradors,' he continues. 'They're quite motivated by food in that when they're feeding they're not too bothered by your presence. When they are chilling out they can often be quite curious though.

We humans seem to be more interesting than plankton, which I'm choosing to take as quite flattering.'

In a nutshell: according to Simon, I have nothing to fear from the whale shark. Correction: almost nothing. They could wipe me out with their tails, he admits, but that is probably all – and even that's avoidable if I follow a few simple rules, such as 'making sure you give them enough space so you're not scaring the shark; meaning it's still able to do its thing.'

'Also,' he adds, 'when people touch them, that can really startle them. Their escape reaction, of course, is to try and get away. They're a huge animal with a very large tail, so they could accidentally hurt someone, but they certainly would never do it on purpose.'

Do not touch, give them space. Oh, and watch their eyes. 'If you are a little bit close and they are a little unsure,' Simon says, 'one of the only vulnerable points on their body is the eye, so you'll see them retract the eye. Almost like the aperture of a camera – they can close it over. Then, if you back off a little, they'll open their eye again.'

Hearing all this first-hand from a smiling whale shark expert, an expert who is alive and not in pieces, I feel a weight inside me start to shift. My interest is deepening. Simon tells me everything I've been dying to know about whale sharks, then adds more. He tells me, for example, that their skin is the thickest of any animal, more than 20 centimetres in some places. He tells me that the male sharks don't have penises but 'claspers', two out-growths located under the pelvic fins, forming the only visible difference between the sexes. He tells me that as-yet-unpublished data from Indonesia is on its way, that researchers out there have managed to track certain whale sharks for more than two years. He tells me that he and his colleagues have no idea how old whale sharks live to, but that he recently saw a juvenile in Tanzania that he first observed eleven years previously. On both occasions, he estimated the shark's length to be the same.

'They are almost certainly growing very slowly,' says Simon. 'I strongly suspect their life expectancy is longer than we think at the moment. For a while we thought it could be between eighty to one hundred, but our best estimate now is about 130.' Then he mentions a Greenland shark that was recently netted as by-catch (i.e. caught non-deliberately by commercial fishing methods). That shark was retinally aged at 397 years old. There's no knowing how much longer it would have lived if it had not been swept up by fishermen. Perhaps the whale shark, similarly, could still surprise us.

Indeed, although Simon has gathered many facts about whale sharks, there is so much more he wants to find out, and not only with regards to their life expectancy. Take the topic of breeding and giving birth. Just thirty or so whale shark pups have ever been found and recorded, says Simon. This from a fish that, as the only recorded pregnant female proved, can carry more than *three hundred* pups in its two uteri during pregnancy, with individual pups at different stages of development within one litter.

'They have the largest litter of any shark,' explains Simon. 'That indicates there would be high mortality, probably, when they're young. It's almost twice as many as any other shark species.' When born, each fish measures 40 to 60 centimetres, making them easy targets. When they are older and larger, on the other hand, the predators become almost non-existent.

Until it comes to their interactions with humans, many of which do not end well for the shark. As you might assume given his official work title (conservation biologist), Simon's biggest preoccupation is conservation: trying to study and mitigate the effects of marine pollution, large-scale fishing, shipping lanes, boat collisions and more. In the seas of Oman, one fishery is known to catch whale sharks for Asian markets such as China, Hong Kong and Thailand, where a single bowl of shark fin soup can cost as much as $100. In other areas, like Pakistan, whale sharks are being netted as by-catch – though whether or not they are then internationally traded is unclear. Meanwhile, in China itself, the largest, most significant whale shark fishery known to the experts has notoriously, and illegally, been threatening the species for years – all for a fin that creates an indistinguishably glutinous texture, and is virtually taste-free. (Mostly it is used to indicate wealth, like flakes of gold leaf sprinkled on a cappuccino.)

'Whale sharks have never been in a worse state than they are now,' says Simon. 'We've probably lost more than half the population.' At the same time, he says, 'whale sharks have never been better protected than they are now, so our job is making sure that this legislative protection actually translates to conservation in action.'

Which makes me wonder what all this means for my aim to swim with the sharks, basking, whale, or otherwise. If boats and pollution are part of the problem, shouldn't I be staying away from these creatures?

Simon replies with an answer I'm not expecting. 'It is the tourism value and interest that has led to whale sharks being protected,' he says, 'and that has led to a few very significant habitats being protected. They're worth tens or hundreds of millions to the global economy.'

Or, to put it another way, a mission like mine could be helping them out long term.

'We have the data to show that if you react in a respectful way with whale sharks – both the whale shark tour operator and the tourists themselves – then it really doesn't affect the whale sharks very much. The whale sharks are in these areas for a reason, and if they can still do what they're there for, then they're not really that bothered by people. If people can go there and have this experience and do something positive for whale shark conservation, I view that as a good thing.'

Before I know it we're on to the juicy info – the Whale Shark Specialist's Top Spots – though they come delivered to me with a disclaimer for transparency: Simon runs trips to some of them to fund research and conservation projects. His advice is that, when it comes to picking an ethical place to find whale sharks, Western Australia is the best. The early operators there were pioneers of eco-tourism, and still carefully restrict the numbers of tourists entering the water at one time. Madagascar, meanwhile, is 'a fairly new hotspot, that's actually progressing really well in terms of management.' The Galapagos, on the other hand, is where Simon saw his biggest whale shark to date. 'It looked like a different species entirely. Literally, the width and size of – and probably heavier than – a single bus. I was just like, *fuck me!*'

In the Philippines, where whale sharks have been protected officially since 1998, Simon recommends Leyte as 'a community-led, proper eco-tourism operation.' It's probably best not to visit Oslob though, he adds, where the locals have been feeding the whale sharks to keep them offshore and bring in the tourist money. 'I don't think the feeding is that great for the sharks,' he explains. 'It's bringing millions to the economy. But the whale sharks are not really being benefitted in my perspective. The education could be so much better, and the money that's being generated isn't really going back into management or conservation or research.'

And what about Georgia Aquarium? Simon says he is currently writing a book with someone who works there. 'I can tell you they really, really care about the whale sharks,' he says. 'They're slightly obsessed by them.'

But still, I say, I think I'd prefer to see them in open ocean.

Simon agrees. Those encounters, he says, are the best.

There is one more spot he recommends for the time of year I'd be able to make a visit – a few months away, in November. He tells me that sightings of juvenile males in this place would effectively be a dead cert at that point in the season. It's an island off the East African coast, apparently – but not one I've heard of before. After I've said my goodbyes and multiple thanks, after my show of gratitude has no doubt started to put Simon on edge, I run to the bus and pull out my phone to look this island up. Its name is Mafia.

I scroll through the pictures online, see a tiny person in snorkelling gear dwarfed by two enormous fish. The whale sharks live there all year round, says one website. 'It has no known connection to organised crime,' says Simon's.

In a bid to finally swim with these massive marine Labradors, I resolve to tap my savings one last time. Either out of pity, or possibly out of interest – the car-crash scene of an ichthyophobe confronting the world's biggest fish – Simon kindly forwards the dates that he'll be there with his colleague, Chris; tells me what flight companies are best; and where he recommends staying. 'Depending on how busy things are for us,' he adds, 'you might be able to come out on our research boat.'

Before I have time to change my mind I book it.

In my haste, I briefly succeed in forgetting the basking sharks. Only when I call Max does it hit home: I now have two supersized challenges to contend with. I'm locked in.

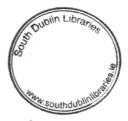

15

Northwest Passage

'Look up, reach up and come up.'

ASCENDING,

PADI OPEN WATER MANUAL, 1999–2007

M uch like Shane on call, Simon has insisted that the best way to encounter basking and whale sharks is not by using air tanks, gauges, computers or BCDs. I don't need to be way down in the sea, says the expert. Instead, if I see them, I need to be able to jump in and keep my cool up near the surface, where they'll be feeding.

'Do you know how to freedive?' he asks me.

'Kind of,' I say, with a creeping dread. 'I can hold my breath for a bit, if that's what you mean.'

'Might be worth looking into,' he replies.

I can't have wasted all this time on scuba practice for nothing. Surely freediving, after that, will be a watery walk in the park, a simple splashing around. This is what I keep telling myself. Until, during a bout of late-morning research – research which begins light and breezy, then morphs into so many internet tabs that my laptop starts to wheeze – I learn a lot more about it. Like how some freedivers will spit blood. Like how long-term practice might permanently injure the brain. Like how some freedivers don't come back from their dives, including one of the world's most celebrated competitors, Natalia Molchova, who vanished without a trace while teaching a private lesson in 2015.

Already I can feel myself deflating. And, at this advanced stage of my quest, this is the last thing I need.

I search for someone, anyone, who can help.

At Hartham Leisure Centre, I meet Adam Drzazga. He's a freediving expert, a previous UK Number One in static apnoea (holding one's breath at the surface), former member of the national freediving team – and runs a freediving school with his freediving wife.

Adam is relentlessly cheerful, and asks if I want to join in. I wondered if he might say this, but today, I've 'forgotten' my swimsuit. Part of me still wants to maintain that the act of freediving is easy. This part wants to observe instead, sitting on the side of the pool in a coat and a thick pair of socks. I can get into the risks and fears from here. Except that Adam has no time for risks and fears.

'Freediving is totally not dangerous,' he tells me. 'Chopping up onions is more dangerous than freediving.'

At least you can chop up onions and still breathe, I think.

Out loud, I ask, 'Are you sure about that?' My mind is stuck on a story, recounted by Max when I told him who I was meeting: about how, back in his school days, a boy at his swimming club drowned in the pool from a blackout while swimming alone. It was rumoured that he'd been practising holding his breath much like freedivers do.

Adam still won't go there. 'Freediving is super extremely peaceful and relaxing,' he says. 'For me, it's as normal as going to Tesco.'

Adam has dived down as far as 78 metres on a single breath – almost a quarter of the distance that Ahmed Gabr descended to on his record-breaking dive, a dive that required about ninety tanks of air. If I wanted to dive more than 60 metres in scuba, PADI tells me I would need to have logged 'a minimum of 175 dives, with at least fifty dives and a hundred hours' experience diving the Type T CCR used in the course with an offboard bailout system. At least twenty-five of these dives must be multistep decompression dives deeper than 40 metres/130 feet with trimix/heliox diluent.' The fact that I can't even translate these statements convinces me that I'm no budding Ahmed. Those depths are out of my league.

With freediving, however, Adam explains, the fact that you take your own breath down with you creates fewer complications. For instance, though the bends is technically possible, it's highly unlikely.

I like the sound of fewer complications. But still, I can't overlook the bends.

'So,' I say. 'It isn't totally safe.'

'Well ...' Adam may be upbeat, but he's also not delusional. As he gets changed, preparing to train with his two students, he finally admits that even he can be nervous when freediving. There is a process involved in the sport, he says. First there is the 'easy phase', during which your last breath is still recent and familiar.

'Then,' says Adam, 'the discomfort starts coming – the carbon dioxide building.' At that point, he tells me, 'I get the two advocates in my head', and with them comes a psychological tussle. 'It's a mental game.' Adam's main priority during this game is to calm the brain and tell it not to panic. Meanwhile the body contracts, desperately seeking air. The brain must overpower the urge to breathe, or the lungs will take in water and cause drowning. Adam mentions times when he's been deep down in the sea, looking up at the distant surface, and feeling that he has no air left: 'a scared moment'.

When that happens, he says, he reminds himself that there are people in place to support him and that he's seconds away from safety. On a deep dive he is attached to a line by a lanyard. Fellow divers vigilantly watch his progress, standing by for accidents. He never freedives alone.

'Back on the surface, your breath is like the first breath you've ever taken in your life.' There are other benefits to freediving, he assures me, aside from this sensation like rebirth. Benefits on top of the fact that it doesn't need lots of equipment, unlike scuba. Benefits like silence. With freediving there are no gas bubbles, no man-made distractions, just the steady pulsing of your heart. Like many freedivers, Adam sees his sport as a form of communion with the sea. He adds that, in nature, blowing bubbles can be interpreted as aggression. Animals have more interest in freedivers, he claims. If you're diving to hunt, for example, you'll catch more fish. Creatures usually come closer then than they would to scuba divers.

I clear my throat. 'So the sharks will be more likely to come up to me?'

As I'm mulling on this, Adam excuses himself. It's time for the more intensive prep to begin. He takes his place on a bench nearby and embarks on twenty minutes of relaxation: holding his breath, slowing his heart rate, closing his eyes, being still. One of his students, Hannah, does likewise, placing noise-cancelling headphones over her ears. I turn to the other, Elliot, a skinny engineering graduate. Is he going to start relaxing too? I ask.

No, he replies. Nothing he can do will lower his heartrate.

He finds the build-up too tense to properly focus. He'll relax when he's in the water.

I ask Elliot why he's here; if he is conquering a phobia too; trying to stimulate calmness in an anxious life; avoiding something more frightening; or, perhaps, simply wanting to swim with big sharks. Turns out it's none of those. Elliot wants to be a merman. A professional merman. One who can charge an hourly rate of £200, and do his thing at pool parties. He tells me he completed a mermaid course in the States. He was only the second man to enrol – the first was an investigative journalist. Now he's on the books of an agency, *listed* as a merman. No one has booked him yet, however. Hartham needs more pool parties. Possibly more pools too.

We talk about the hazards that freediving involves, and Elliot shares his belief that all trainee freedivers should experience an underwater blackout, as long as there's a pro nearby to help. It's a controversial opinion, and his teacher disagrees ('A blackout *isn't* something you seek or want'). But, in a way, Elliot's high-risk tactic fits with what I've been learning. Consider the worst. Gain knowledge. The same message, again and again.

Elliot, Hannah and Adam rest on the tiles. They enter the pool in their wetsuits. Previous complaints from other swimmers mean that their school must hire its own lane for these sessions: the locals were suspicious of the divers swimming beneath them. As the freedivers get themselves ready, I watch a member of the public swim a few lengths. She is wearing long diamanté earrings, the kind you might put on for a cocktail soirée. The sparkly tips of them drag in the chlorine. Is *this* not suspicious behaviour?

Meanwhile, in the freediving corner, Hannah and Adam are on their backs, lying face-up in the water. Elliot stands between them, counting down aloud from the three-minute mark. During the last thirty seconds, Adam appears to be hoovering air, churning his lips like a baby wanting to suckle or start crying. At zero, Elliot turns them both over, down into the pool. Then, with gestures not unlike those one might ascribe to a Deep Southern pastor, Elliot keeps a hand on each of their backs, reassuringly presiding over this weird, wonky, leisure centre baptism. His touch stops them drifting, or knocking against the side.

Each freediver lies submerged for as long as they can, two faceless figures bobbing. Long after Hannah turns over, Adam is still going. His floating dreadlocks have turned into stalks of rockweed.

'Five minutes, thank you,' says Elliot, watching the clock, unexpectedly polite. 'Thank you, five minutes thirty.' Maybe the *thank yous* are meant to create a safe sense of banality, of ordinariness, in this scene. But it's jarring. I think I see Adam convulse. His body seems tense. So does mine. 'Six minutes, thank you,' says Elliot.

Nothing about what's unfolding here feels ordinary. I'm convinced that I'm about to witness a blackout. Then, at six minutes and fifteen seconds, Adam puts his arms to the side of the pool and begins to bring himself round. At six minutes thirty, he finally draws breath.

'Are you having fun?' he asks me, seconds later.

'Yeah!' I shout from the side of the pool, though *fun* is not quite the word. *A traumatic-hypnotic episode* would be more accurate. 'You?' I ask.

'Yeah!' Adam shouts. 'Absolutely!'

Later, when Adam is taking a break, I ask him what went through his mind during those minutes underwater.

'For four minutes I was lying there dead,' he says. 'After, the breath work starts.' Then the mental arguments began. 'It's such a brain-fucking thing,' he says. 'You have to find one positive why you should not stop. Because there are ten reasons why you should.'

I feel like I know what he means.

Too soon, I'm packing to go to the Hebrides. Mentally I am not ready. Even after talking to Shane and Simon. Even after Adam assures me I'll have a great time without tanks. Even though I'm not yet heading for the biggest fish in the sea. And even though Max has spent every day for the past two weeks reminding me how lucky I am to be going.

'It's the trip of a lifetime,' he tells me. 'Followed by *another* trip of a lifetime!'

'Join me,' I say for the umpteenth time since he arrived back at mine for the evening.

He shakes his head. 'You said you wanted to do it alone, remember?'

'That's what I feel I *ought* to do. Not what I *want* to do.'

'Well, it's done now. And I wouldn't have been able to get off work anyway.' He smiles, sympathetically, then grabs me by the shoulders, trying to shake his enthusiasm into me. 'Trip. Of. A *lifetime.*'

As I zip up my washbag, I feel myself stalling. I break off to breathe. Then I call Mandi, my friend and sage who took part in the Oxford CBT study to cure her arachnophobia. Maybe she has some more insights to impart, more helpful nuggets she picked up from the professionals.

'In Thailand, after I'd done my training, I probably could have swum with a whale shark,' I relay to her. 'I think I was just about prepped. But thinking about any fish now is starting to freak me out again.'

'Yeah,' replies Mandi. 'Actually, me and the spiders aren't going that well either . . . '

Mandi tells me she didn't keep up the things that she

learned during the CBT study. She didn't practise. She tells me that she can't deal with spiders any more. That her husband has to kill them before she can relax. If she was asked to walk up to a tarantula in a tank now, she thinks her reactions would be back to square one.

'I know that if I made myself sit with the panic and look at spiders again – you know, like, faced my fear – eventually I'd feel fine. But that process, well . . . It's just so horrible. I really don't want to. And it's fine most of the time anyway. I mean, it's an issue in September, when they come back into the house. And I know I could never visit Australia because there are spiders *everywhere*. But apart from that it's bearable. I can live with it.

'You need a decent motivation to stick with fighting a phobia,' says Mandi. 'I just don't have it. Do you?'

On dark streets I start my journey, alone. Max will have fallen asleep as soon as I left, recharging for his next day in the office. I, meanwhile, am taking the Caledonian Sleeper from Euston up to Glasgow. There I'll change stations and head to my fate on the coast.

For the time being, rather than worrying about big fish or death, I transfer my worries to thoughts of missing various travel connections. The change in focus gives me some relief, and I board the sleeper, ready to rest in the style that the service suggests. But sleep, of course, won't come.

No one could reach Coll from London by accident. The journey is a quest unto itself. After pulling into Glasgow the next morning, uncoiling from the cold angst-ball of my body, I grind through the city to warm up and change stations, pump my legs against an icy seat, keep my tired eyes glued to departures, then board a three-hour train service to the end of the line at Oban.

The train lurches towards stations with make-believe names

like Loch Awe and Falls of Cruachan. Grassy hilltops glow in the morning light. At one point I look up to see a graveyard of boats at Bowling Harbour – wrecks in various states of decay – and I watch the scene wondering if this is some sort of omen.

Oban itself, when we get there, is dour in the drizzle. I walk to my hostel along the seafront, watching the rain-swathed islands out on the bay – Kerrera, Lismore, Mull. Tomorrow I have an early start to catch the first ferry to Coll. In the meantime, I have several hours to explore the town on my own.

It is the Friday of the August bank holiday, not that you could tell it from the temperature – these breezes, fresh from the Atlantic, are completely nipple-stiffening. Tourists gather nonetheless, here to hop the islands. It seems to me that every couple in Scotland is out in force today: beaming holidaymakers, cheered by the water, wrapping each other up in their arms, brandishing matching raincoats against the grey. Unable to nestle in anyone else's shadow, missing Max and his optimism, I zip up my collar and walk by the beach, looking for clues to sharks out in the water. A rope of kelp. A crushed plastic bottle. A stranded jellyfish glinting like a flattened crystal ball.

An active gull next to the sea wall catches my eye. My approach scares it away from a toddler-sized chunk of blubber. Never before have I seen blubber in the flesh, so to speak. This piece is grey and odourless, and two small bones poke from its side. I kneel down to better judge what it came from. A whale, perhaps. A dolphin. A person. Leaning closer, I see small hairs on its surface; a scattering of dark speckles. Seal. It must be seal. But how did it come to be here? Orca attack? Hungry shark? Another omen, either way.

I take a picture and send it to Max. 'Found some dead seal on the beach,' I write. 'Wish you were here.'

'Sounds like you're having a brill time,' he replies.

*

My alarm the next morning is set for 5.05. In the run-up, I doze on my hostel bunk in a semi-fevered state. I have visions of missing the boat by ten minutes, reaching the ferry terminal to see it steaming into the Sound of Mull, a horny Canadian staring me down with a vengeful grin on his face. In fact, I wake as soon as my phone vibrates, and spring from the bed more alert in mind than my body has the energy to support. The result is a messy stumbling to the shower, where I flinch beneath its painful jets of water.

Washed and dressed with time to spare, I hoick on my gear and march out to the moonlit streets of Oban. I've gone about 5 metres up the road when a woman's voice calls out to me from a parked taxi.

'You heading for the ferry terminal?'

'Yes.'

'So are we. Want a lift?'

Inside the taxi I find Kay and Sam, a mother and her adult son from Yorkshire. Kay says they have travelled from Edinburgh, where Sam studies, and now they are travelling over to Coll on the ferry.

'Me too,' I reply. 'I'm supposed to be swimming with basking sharks.'

'So are we,' says Kay. 'But have you seen the weather for tomorrow? It really doesn't look good. The whole week doesn't really.'

'Ah.'

'It doesn't look good,' she repeats.

I ask them if they're scared of finding the basking sharks.

Kay frowns. She looks at her son, then looks back at me, clearly bemused by the question. 'Nah,' she says.

'Nah,' says Sam. It really does sound like they mean it.

We part ways on the ferry and I watch for passing basking sharks from a corner of the rear deck. The sea is calm, far calmer than I had expected, so any tall dorsal fins should be easy to spot. But apart from a small group of porpoises, who slink through the waves by Loch Linnhe, the water keeps its secrets to itself.

I think back to that 100 per cent success figure, unable to believe that I am really going to see the second largest fish in the whole world. How can I be that sure I am about to swim with one? It seems unfathomable that any sharks should be here; that this is something which can be done off the British coast, simply by taking two trains and a ferry. Unfathomable that giant sharks could be this accessible. To me, of all people.

My brain flicks back through its cache of photos and videos; its memories of fear and fish bites. By the time we're docking on the Isle of Coll, I've worked myself up into a fierce state of anticipation. While the crew paves the way for us to disembark, I receive a message from a colleague of Simon Pierce who, strangely enough, came out on this same trip last week. When I contacted him, he promised to update me on his progress. The update reads: 'We didn't see anything on the first day, but the second was very productive and we jumped in with five different sharks! The third day we were beaten by the weather.'

Five sharks. Five. And that was during a three-day tour, not a four-day tour like mine.

This is really happening, I think. *I'm going to do this. I'm going to swim with a giant shark. Going to swim with a giant unknown.*

Though it looks like I'm not going to swim with it tomorrow. After gathering up the three- and four-dayers from the ferry terminal car park – sixteen prospective shark-seekers in total – the tour organisers drop us off at the island's community centre for a welcome briefing. Kay's bleak weather predictions are confirmed.

'It's looking like it'll be pretty stormy,' says Gillian, our

Scottish-American guide. 'Not great conditions for being on the boat. I'm sorry. We might put on a lecture or something, maybe do a snorkel trip from the land.'

Disappointed murmurs fill the hall.

'It is a really good day for weather today, though,' she continues, 'and we've another group out now on their last trip. They'll be back at five, and then we're planning to take you guys on the water for a few hours from six o'clock. If they see sharks today, we'll go looking for them. How does that sound?'

Excitement ripples through the room. *Today. We could be swimming with sharks* today.

After having our wetsuit measurements checked, we're released to while away the hours however we wish. I want to keep my eyes on the water, gain a better sense of what I'm getting into, so I borrow a pair of binoculars, buy biscuits from a tiny shop, and make my way to the nearest beach. The weather must be superb for shark-spotting. It's bright and warm and windless. I feel certain that, while I walk on this single-track road, an offshore assortment of landlubbers is blowing their minds in the presence of British sea monsters.

There are no dorsal fins for me at Cliad Bay – not much sign of marine life at all, apart from seabirds and kelp. After pacing the sand in bare feet, I lie down by a sheltered dune and cover my face with my shirt. The waves recede from my ears.

A blank patch follows. I'm shocked awake by a chatting trio of walkers strolling by. I sit bolt upright and check my watch: have I missed the boat? No, there are still hours to go. My eyes readjust to the sunshine. Preparing to get to my feet, I am brushing the sand from my hair when a solid, dark shape appears in the shallows.

I grab the binoculars, and desperately peer through the finders, trying to blink past the sight of my own eyelashes.

Then, boom, up it comes: the head of a common seal. So much like a person. Not so much like a shark. It must be about 100 metres from me, and seems to have no idea it's being watched. I follow it with the binoculars, then lose sight of it behind a cluster of wet rocks.

Back at the island's bunkhouse, where I and most of the shark-seekers are staying, the suspense is steadily mounting. Kay is fixed to the local weather forecast, refreshing the relevant web page again and again.

'It's not getting any better for tomorrow,' she reports. 'And our last day looks bad too. *Your* last day looks all right though,' she tells me. 'Probably the best day of the trip.' She puts down her phone. 'I'll be gutted if we don't see them.'

I share with her what Shane told me on the phone: that the sharks are definitely here; that we only need the right weather; if just part of one day is fine we'll see them.

'Could be tonight,' I say. But the truth is I have my doubts. If I can travel to Koh Bon and be one of only four divers *not* to witness the massive manta ray, if I can spend weeks in whale shark territory without a single glimpse, surely I can travel to Coll and curse a whole boatload of people. Perhaps I've spent too much time wishing fish away. This is the result.

At six, we make our way to the pier and split into two groups. Settling down in the seat beside me is Alison, a diver who has travelled to Coll from Surrey.

'If we don't see any sharks on this trip it could be my fault,' she confesses. 'I once spent £3000 on a storm-chasing tour through the States. Not one drop of rain the whole holiday.'

I smile. I've found an ally.

On the other side of our boat is a pair of Spanish twins with giant cameras. They speak in whispered tones to each other, existing in a private world of their own. At the front, a family of four are poised – mother, father, son and his girlfriend – all decked out in their own gear. Behind me stands a guy called Mike, who runs sea kayaking trips from his home on the mainland. There are also two guides, plus a volunteer wildlife spotter. And, of course, the skipper.

I count them up. Twelve. With me, we're lucky thirteen.

Swatting at midges, guide Luke welcomes us all and begins his intro. The boat pulls away from the pier.

'Bad news is that we're *definitely* not going out on the water tomorrow,' Luke confirms. 'Good news is we've just come back from a trip to Gunna Sound, which is just down the west coast here. And we had some really great shark encounters there today. So that's where we're going to head now, OK? See if the sharks are still there. They can appear anywhere, though, so keep watching the sea and shout if you see anything.'

My body feels rock-heavy in the seat.

'Want to get into your wetsuit, Georgie?'

As we speed down the coast I pull on my swimming gear, catching my throat in the suit's twisted hood. Nobody is saying it, but I'm certain we're all wondering who will jump in with the sharks first. There are rules, Luke reminds us as we go. Only four can be in the water with a shark at any one time. There must be no diving beneath the shark. No touching the shark. No interfering with the shark whatsoever. I can hardly believe these instructions are being given to a group that includes me. More disbelief comes when I realise what I'm thinking: *I don't want to wait any more. I want to go first.*

Minutes later there's a shout, but it's a false alarm. A harbour porpoise is swimming gracefully, at a distance from the boat. We can't get in with those, Luke tells us: it's against UK law to deliberately try to swim with cetaceans (whales, dolphins and porpoises – the aquatic mammals). They're too intelligent. Too likely to be affected by our being there.

'Are you telling us basking sharks are idiots?' says Alison.

Luke breaks off from scanning the waves. 'They've got very small brains,' he says.

I ask whether anyone on his tours is ever afraid of fish. 'Not really,' he replies. 'Sharks, sometimes, but fish no. I've had more people on trips who were scared of the water. There was one woman who could get her body in but not her face. She spent ages with it about a centimetre away from the surface, just staring down, like she couldn't break the barrier. I had to encourage her on the whole time, but once she got it in she was like, "Oh!"' He makes a noise of pleasant surprise. 'When we got her swimming with the sharks, she loved it.

'They *can* look pretty scary, though,' he adds. 'With their mouths closed they look amazingly similar to a great white, only they're *much* bigger.'

Oh God.

Fully suited and wetsuit-booted, I huddle up to the gang of voyagers keeping eyes peeled for new fins. A line of black pierces upwards through a wave.

'Ah!' I cry. 'Over there!'

Several pairs of eyes switch to where I'm pointing: straight at the neck of a guillemot. I apologise. Another false alarm.

As we continue our approach to the shark zone, we hear more about what happened earlier in Luke's day. How his group spent an uneventful morning on the water, until their fortunes changed. Waves of plankton in the sound brought the large fish to the surface, he says – not only sharks, but an ocean sunfish too, the glove-like creature that grows to around 2.5 metres tall from fin to fin. One of the basking sharks, he says, was 8 metres in length. Just its dorsal fin alone was 1 metre in height. That's a fin which would span from the floor to my hip. I cannot believe we are talking about a real creature.

We arrive at Gunna Sound, a stretch of water between the south of Coll and its neighbouring island, Tiree. Our skipper eases off the engines. It's time for slow cruising, all eyes open and primed. Conversation rises and falls like the motions of the waves. We see another porpoise. More seabirds. Then I overhear Mike, the sea kayaker, telling Alison he came on this same trip before.

'Just don't ask me what I saw,' he says, his tone conveying an audible grimace.

'Or what you didn't see, eh?' chuckles Alison.

'You did this trip before?' I interject. 'And you didn't see any sharks?'

Mike looks at me and says nothing. Meanwhile I am calculating what this means for the luck of our boat. Maybe *Mike* is the cursed one . . .

'There!' someone shouts. 'No, wait – it's just a bird.'

We loop around Gunna Sound for over two hours. The group's posture changes gradually, from upright to loose, sleepy. Raincoats go over wetsuits, fending off the chill. I want to stop looking and rest but I can't. When the shark comes I want to know. I want to be ready.

Eventually the light begins to fade. 'We're going to make our way home to the pier now,' says Luke. 'The sharks must have followed the plankton back down the water column.'

But having psyched myself up so thoroughly to see sharks, I still cling to the idea of seeing something – a flash of fin, an open jaw – before we dock back on the island. I cannot peel my eyes away from the water, nor bring myself to strip out of my wetsuit. Even then, as hard as I stare, I don't spot what the skipper sees.

'Bottlenose dolphins,' he announces. 'Ten o'clock.'

Great, I think. *More dolphins*. But I stand up and watch with the rest of the boat nevertheless. Moments later, my gaze alights on a gathering of serpentine shapes. They are cleaving through the water, perhaps 50 metres from us. When our boat slows the animals change their course and head in our direction. These creatures are huge, far bigger than the dolphins I encountered in New Zealand. Judging by the time it takes them to rise up and slip away, one of the pod, a grey adult covered in scars, must be over 3 metres long.

They trail us, slither over each other, appear in unexpected patches of water. One bursts out right next to me, and I clutch my chest in shock. I've no idea how I could cope swimming with this. But watching their powerful, brawny forms from the deck, accompanied by the delighted whoops of the group is – well – exhilarating. The other boat arrives to watch them too, and I see Kay and Sam on the back of it, framed by a glowing supermoon. It's a surreal scene. And an eerie one. But a good omen. Surely good.

True to everyone's forecasts, the weather the following morning is abysmal. Rain and driving winds contort the trees outside our windows with gusts of up to 45 miles per hour. After a brisk walk to wake myself up and check that, yes, the weather is really that bad, I pick up a local book about basking shark hunting: *Hebridean Sharker,* by Tex Geddes.

In it, Geddes, a Scottish author-adventurer, describes how he sought to revive the shark liver oil industry in the 1950s, equipping a boat with guns and harpoons and patrolling the Scottish west coast. His account reads like a macho, romanticised view of destruction: enormous sharks shot and pulled aboard, the ages and efforts it takes to kill them, livers cut out while the sharks are still breathing, the rest of the animal tossed back into the sea. Hardy men muck in with the slaughter and joke, posing for photographs next to their weapons, revelling in their own strength. Sometimes they even dip into the shark oil to sharpen up their suntans. Every few pages I have to stop. Geddes' throwaway violence is hurting my eyes.

A morning presentation, delivered by Luke, continues on this theme, retelling the gory history of the basking sharks. In peak times, he reports, Norwegians killed more than four thousand baskers a year in this area, adding to the numbers annually wiped out by the Scots until the final basking shark to be hunted here twitched its last in 1994. A shark's liver forms 25 per cent of a basking shark's bodyweight, Luke informs us. It was highly sought after for its purported health-boosting benefits; for its use in industrial lubricants; as an ingredient in perfumes and cosmetics, and so on. Their rough skin was also sold – a tough form of leather that cuts when stroked the wrong way – while their bones were ground to make fertiliser.

Luke takes us back and across to Canada in the fifties, where a particularly gruesome extermination project had apparently permanent consequences for the basking shark population. The Canadian sharks were not exterminated because they were dangerous to humans – they weren't at all (Tex Geddes describes them as being so tame that a crew mate could throw an anchor into one's mouth) – but because the great size of the shark would damage the fishermen's gear if they swam into it. Luke shows us a poster depicting a boat equipped with a large, sharp blade on its prow. It was designed to be rammed into the fish, to slice the basking sharks in half, causing instant death for death's sake, with no subsequent harvesting of oil or bones or leather. The project was so successful that the 'pests' were just about decimated. Their numbers have never recovered.

In this part of Britain, however, and at this time of year, basking sharks still gather in huge numbers. Luke tells us the sharks are everywhere around us. They are in these waters *right now*, without a doubt. In August 2012, he explains, a plane flew over the area to complete a visual survey. The spotter counted 918 basking sharks in one day. And those were just the ones that were visibly feeding off blooms of plankton. It's thought that the sharks only do this for 10 per cent of their lives. The rest of the time they are filtering food underwater.

Luke tells us that, while its mouth is large, the basking shark's throat is small; that the shark would be physically unable to swallow us. He tells us that they usually swim at a speed of about two knots. He tells us that, sometimes, the basking sharks breach, leaping full out of the water and flopping back into the waves. He tells us they can show fear-like behaviour. That they will dive or swim away quickly if threatened. That, as well as having human predators, they can also be prey for groups of devious orcas.

When the lecture is over I feel like I know basking sharks better than ever. I feel like this knowledge will get me through. Help me stay calm in the water. I also feel horribly culpable. The violations Luke described seem to form compelling evidence of what can happen when something living (a human, a fish, a shark) is reduced to no more than a concept (a source of income, a pest). And isn't that what I've been doing? For years now I've been turning fish into something abstract and other: fear, danger, death, the unknown. What I still haven't done is accepted what they are. Accepted that they are different. And that their difference is not intrinsically negative.

In the latest official summary of worldwide shark attacks – the 2017 analysis of data compiled by the International Shark Attack File (ISAF) – 155 shark-on-human attacks were recorded in one year. Of these, eighty-eight were classed as unprovoked; 'incidents where an attack on a live human occurs in the shark's natural habitat, with no human provocation of the shark.' Thirty of the rest were classed as provoked: the result of grabbing a shark, attempting to fish it, etc. The remaining thirty-seven were a mix of other classifications, including attacks in public aquaria (one), attacks on marine vessels rather than people (eighteen), and 'doubtful' attacks, that were most likely misreported, involving no shark at all (twelve).

Of all these 155 attacks, the majority of the victims (59 per cent) were involved in surfing or some kind of board-sport at the time. Just three of the number were scuba diving. More importantly, only five of the whole year's attacks proved to be fatal.

As the ISAF puts it, 'The worldwide total number of unprovoked shark attacks is remarkably low given the billions of people participating in aquatic recreation every year ... By contrast about 100 million sharks and rays are killed each year by fisheries.'

That's twenty million sharks and rays for each human fatality.

The figure makes my brain ache, whichever way I look at it, and doesn't even account for the billions of other sea creatures killed year on year. The numbers mean that, on average, over three sharks and rays were killed *every second* during 2017. On a night where I slept seven hours, there would have been almost eighty thousand fewer sharks living by the time I ate my toast the next morning than there had been when I laid my head on the pillow. Some of those caught will have been basking sharks. Some, as I know from Simon, will have been whale sharks.

And whereas the fish most people fear, the carnivorous sharks – great whites, tigers, bulls and the like – are highly efficient killers that leave very little to waste, our fishermen employ tactics against them that, were they to be used against humans, would be classed not only as sociopathic, but extraordinarily excessive. Longlines of baited hooks indiscriminately catch anything that swims past, sometimes stretching more than 60 miles through the sea. Hanging from hooks, these sharks thrash and struggle. The fish that can't take in oxygen without any forward movement drown on the line. But perhaps it is better to drown than the alternative: a fisherman dragging you out of the water, slicing off your fins to be sold, then throwing your now-useless body back into the sea, letting you bleed to death on the sandy floor.

The truth I need to face up to is that fish do not exist to scare land mammals like myself. For millions of years, before humans even existed, before even the existence of trees, they have sat at the top of the ocean food chain, weeding out unhealthy marine life and sustaining the overall balance of eco-systems. Without sharks, smaller herbivore-eaters flourish, the herbivores themselves decline in number and algae growth is left unchecked, meaning less space and fewer resources for life-giving reefs. The effect of shark intimidation in grassy areas also stops ocean herbivores overgrazing. In turn, this prevents the collapse of habitats. And helps the sea do what it has done for aeons: regulate the carbon dioxide released into our atmosphere.

But the myths we have built around sharks have led to butchery and imbalance. We've allowed ourselves to hold on to fear and disgust. Antagonists, after all, can be such a thrill. They give us purpose, stimulation, something defined to conquer. And given what we've done to them over the years, what we continue to do to the shark population alone, surely we could forgive these creatures for occasionally fighting back. Surely retaliation would be justified. Yet the fish have not set out to destroy humanity. According to these statistics, rarely does any shark strike one of our own.

I remember reading Thor Heyerdahl's account of his 1947 Kon-Tiki expedition, a journey across the currents from Peru to Polynesia. What stood out for me was the moment they met a 'veritable sea monster'.

Knut [Haugland — the raft's radio operator] had been squatting there, washing his pants in the swell, and when he looked up for a moment he was staring straight into the biggest and ugliest face any of us had ever seen in the whole of our lives. It was the head of a veritable sea monster, so huge and hideous that, if the Old Man of the Sea himself had come up, he could not have made such an impression on us.

The description continues.

The monster came quietly, lazily swimming after us from astern. It grinned like a bulldog and lashed gently with its tail . . . When the giant came close up to the raft, it rubbed its back against the heavy steering oar, which was just lifted up out of the water, and now we had ample opportunity of studying the monster at the closest quarters — at such close quarters that I thought we had all gone mad . . . Walt Disney himself, with all his powers of imagination, could not have created a more hair-raising sea monster than that which thus suddenly lay with its terrific jaws along the raft's side.

It turns out this was a whale shark, and, to Thor Heyerdahl and his crew, it appeared 'so grotesque, inert and stupid . . . that we could not help shouting with laughter, although we realized that it had strength enough in its tail to smash both balsa logs and ropes to pieces if it attacked us.'

But the whale shark did not attack them. Instead Heyerdahl recounts how it circled the raft for about an hour until a member of his crew, Erik Hesselberg, the raft's navigator, found its visit 'too exciting' and 'thrust [his] harpoon with all his giant strength down between his legs and deep into the whale shark's gristly head. It was a second or two before the giant understood what was happening. Then in a flash the placid half-wit was transformed into a mountain of steel muscles . . . [The] giant stood on its head and plunged down into the depths . . . We waited a long time for the monster to come racing back like an infuriated submarine, but we never saw anything more of him.'

It's tempting to say, 'These guys wrote in a different time. People didn't know better back then.' But the killing is still happening, partly because us humans are still afraid, partly because we don't know any better, partly because we don't see the need to change. *I* need to change.

I try again with Tex Geddes. This time I learn that basking sharks can sometimes be smelt before they are seen. I wonder if it will be my nose that signals my first encounter here. I attempt to read more but am losing my stomach for killing, so opt to take refuge in the common room of the bunkhouse. The book stays where it is.

Two ladies from the three-day boat, a friendly pair from Sussex called Emma and Nat, are lounging on the sofa, driven by boredom to have a go at a 208-piece jigsaw. As we get to talking over cups of tea, I discover that Emma works as a specialist in cognitive behavioural therapy. I slam down my cup and lean forward.

'You're exactly what I've been missing.'

Emma laughs, then glances at Nat.

'Seriously,' I say, 'CBT is why I'm here. Well, kind of.'

I explain about my fish phobia; about learning to scuba dive; about how I got the idea from Mandi; how my fears of fish seem to ebb and flow; how I can't get a handle on them.

'I need to get on with my life,' I say. 'I should be spending time with my boyfriend this weekend, I should be saving, there's so many other things I ought to deal with instead, but I'm chasing after fish, chucking my money at them. I can't properly focus on anything else. It's all fish, fish, fish and fear, fear, fear.' Emma listens, puzzle piece in hand, and nods along with professional patience.

When I pause to draw a new breath, she tells me she works with phobics regularly, and that CBT treatment can be extremely effective for them. But, she says, it needs to be done properly.

I dread to ask after all this time, but better late than never. 'What do you class as properly? I mean, what's the best way of getting rid of a phobia for good?'

'Repeat, repeat, repeat,' Emma says. 'Learn all about what you're scared of. Read about it, watch films, look for articles.'

'I've been doing that.'

'Good,' Emma replies. 'But you need to keep going. If you stop working towards that goal, there's time to let the fear build again.' She talks about phobias like a gardener talks about weeds: you need to get rid of every last root or those pesky things will come back. 'If there's even the tiniest bit of avoidance left it won't go away,' she explains.

Laying down her puzzle piece, Emma then introduces me to the 'Anxiety Equation', helping me to scrawl it into my notebook:

$$Anxiety = \frac{Likelihood \times Awfulness}{Rescue + Ability\ to\ Cope}$$

Likelihood, she tells me, is the chance that the phobia will come true. In case it does come true, *Awfulness* is the answer to, 'What's the worst that could possibly happen?' *Ability to Cope* is a person's confidence in their own abilities to ride out that phobia. And *Rescue* is the support that others might offer when shit hits the fan.

Emma shares a common example. A theoretical patient, let's call her Hilda, turns up for CBT sessions because she is afraid of driving; because driving triggers major anxieties for her. Emma will ask Hilda what exactly about driving she is afraid of.

'That I will come off the road and kill lots of people,' Hilda says.

'What's the *likelihood* of that happening? Emma will ask. 'Has it happened to you before?' She might help Hilda to look up statistics, such as how many people drive every day versus how many people come off the road and kill people.

Next, the *awfulness*: how terrible would it be if that accident happened?

'Pretty awful,' says Hilda. 'The worst thing in my life.'

And that might well be the truth. But the equation is not over. Next, Emma will ask Hilda to imagine other people in her nightmare car crash scenario, people who might be able to offer *rescue*. She explains that many phobics imagine dealing with fears on their own. But in the case of a traffic disaster, for instance, there will be other people getting out of their cars around the scene, offering support, calling paramedics and policemen to help further. Later, there may be family and friends. Or even therapists, like Emma.

Lastly, she will ask Hilda how she would *cope* with this awful event.

'Really badly,' Hilda might say.

'But how?' Emma will press.

Together, they will look at examples of times when Hilda has dealt with other traumatic events. What she did. How she reacted. Hilda must have got through these things one way or another, or she would not still be here to tell the tale.

The trick of this equation is to minimise the power of what's on the top (i.e. likelihood and awfulness), and max-imise the size of what's on the bottom (rescue and coping abilities). Sometimes, according to Emma, a mere six sessions will set someone on the right path. But that patient also needs to practise alone, gradually increasing their own exposure, and keeping up the momentum.

'I need to up my exposure to the fish I don't know then,' I conclude. 'The giant ones especially.'

'Yep,' says Emma. 'Swimming with them every day would be ideal.'

I look back out of the window at the thick sheets of rain being whipped past the glass, heavy water cascading all over the church, the grass and the fences. With hundreds of mas-sive sharks in the seas around us, Coll could be the perfect place for my therapy. If only the gales would subside.

After lunch, heeding my wishes, the wind dies down a little. Although the rain continues to fall, cabin fever forces me out in my waterproofs. I may not be able to swim yet, but I can still up my exposure to the sea. I walk along the harbour to the pier, passing a freestanding cast of a giant whale's jaw-bones. There is still no sign of fins in the surf, but beneath me a seal pokes its puppy-like face out of the water, then disappears.

Continuing up a boggy path, I reach the next stretch of coastline. Shafts of sunlight halo the waves. I look again for dorsal fins, and, while I'm standing on the beach, I realise that I'm being watched myself. Another dark head is peering out from the bay. Another seal. I stay where I am, motionless, and watch it watching me. The seal dips down. Then a second head appears. And a third. When I blink, they disappear.

Yesterday Luke told us how basking sharks will sometimes enter the shallows to find plankton. I feel sure that at some point or another, perhaps on multiple occasions, a shark will have drifted into this stretch of water right here, or possibly more than one shark – a school, a shoal, a shiver. If I could stand here long enough, keeping my eyes on the prize, I know, I am certain, that I would see one eventually.

As if it is able to read my mind, a seal pops back up at the surface. With a raised nose, it points its head skyward. The pose creates a solid, dark triangle, exactly like the triangle of a shark fin. Moments later, its nose comes back down: I'm being watched again. Then another seal head appears. Now the two of them tip back their noses. *Two* dorsal fins. It looks like they're trying to tell me something. I wonder if this is some kind of Skippy situation – and they've both seen something I've missed. *What's that, Sealy? A basking shark? There? In the water?* My eyes search wildly across the bay. But there aren't any real fins around them. Only the two of them tilting their heads.

Are they actually taking the piss?

The next morning I pull on my wetsuit without needing to be prompted. I have knowledge. I have a group of people who can rescue me. And I am impatient. I want to continue along this journey of fearlessness. I want to gear myself up for the whale shark.

Soon after greeting us on the boat, Luke announces that 'This is perfect shark-spotting weather.' We are pulling out of the harbour, and a large pair of binoculars is bolted to his face.

'I'm very confident we'll see basking sharks today,' he

continues. 'Not too sunny, so no glare. Calm water. The fins will stick out really clearly in this.'

At Gunna Sound the signs are still right. Luke points out a froth of surface plankton. It marks the line of the tide, and should be a basking shark magnet. We pass beside it, expecting to see the three tell-tale tips of a basker: the tail fin, the dorsal fin and the peak of its open mouth as it's feeding. When Gillian, our second guide, calls, 'Shark!' I think, *This is it*, but she cannot fix on what she saw and now it has disappeared.

'Might have been something else,' she murmurs.

The skipper takes us on a big loop around the eastern side of the bay, and I feel again like someone who has booked to see a performance but turned up late – right after the show closed to go on tour. The feeling isn't helped by some of Luke's stories – the aggregation of fifty sharks they saw just a few weeks ago, for example. I also discover that Mike, the kayaker who did this trip once before, was joking about not seeing sharks on his first go. In fact he saw between ten and fifteen on the same bank holiday weekend. He swam with them several times.

'It was amazing,' he says. 'At one point, Luke and I were snorkelling, and this huge shark swam right underneath us. I've got that image frozen in my mind.'

Each new tale makes me more expectant, and more nervous. They are here. They are *here*. And so am I. But the water seems too choppy. It has too much swell.

Luke parts from his binoculars for a moment and says, 'Without these waves around us right now we'd be seeing shark fins for sure.' I want to spit.

Eventually, he suggests we try out our gear on a short swim with the seals. 'Make sure everything's good for when the sharks come.'

I have never swum with seals but I've heard stories about

their viciousness. One contact told me about his time in Antarctica, where it was widely known that a leopard seal had attacked a young diving biologist. It dragged her in to be drowned. 'Leopard seals are massive things though,' he'd added. 'Not like the ones you'll find up there in Scotland.'

As the skipper pulls into a spot by the bay, there are seal heads all around us. Leopard or not, they look big enough to me. Still, I'm aware that I can't put off getting into the sea around here for ever. Luke issues the instructions – don't drift out of his sight, be careful of the current, try not to splash if you want to see anything – and because I'm already in my gear, primed to rip the plaster off my shark-shaped wound, I'm among the first group of swimmers to disembark. Unfortunately I am also the slowest – floating so high I'm mostly kicking air; unnaturally buoyant because of the extra-thick suit I've hired to protect me from the cold. I soon start slipping behind.

Yielding to my lagging status, I peer through my mask and stare into the water. A thickly growing kelp forest bows beneath the waves, hiding who knows what. Tiny, brown-coloured organisms – some kind of plankton, I'm guessing – bob in every direction. And there are jellyfish, unreal jellyfish, with delicate lines of coloured lights that flicker down their sides. It is as if I'm inside a Scottish-themed episode of *Blue Planet*, and thanks to the gloves and hood I am borrowing, I feel as immune from being stung as if I was watching this scene play out from my sofa.

Torn between wanting to catch up with the group and knowing I need to minimise my splashing, I begin to swim with my arms alone; a slow breaststroke. Grey shapes form in the corner of my eye and I turn to see them better, but they flicker like weak holograms, shimmering through a haze of floating nutrients. They are seals drawn on tracing paper.

I try to look harder, to bring them into focus, but they're too distant.

I look back up out of the water. My fellow swimmers all have their faces immersed. I cannot tell what they are seeing, or if they are seeing anything. And to keep the seals around us I must be quiet. We all must be quiet. I look down into the water again. Now it is just me, the kelp, the plankton and the disco-style jellyfish. A school of small sand eels wiggles past, risking their lives away from their natural habitat.

In the very next instant, the biggest seal I've ever seen passes right under my body, no more than 3 metres beneath me. It is broad and long – the size of a man, albeit a short one – and stares up at me intently as it swims. Its eyes are so wide I can see the whites. It must be seeing the same of me through my mask. This seal looks disconcertingly muscular. I've no doubt it could overpower me in a moment. But it doesn't. Instead it leads its wide eyes on and melts into the murk. I float for a second, assessing my reaction to what just happened. The verdict: speeding heartbeat, shaking joints, but not full panic mode. As if undergoing its own CBT course, aware of Emma's advice – *repeat, repeat, repeat* – the big seal then passes under me once again. I cannot tear my eyes from it, and not only because I want to be prepped to defend myself. It's the shimmer of the seal, the dazzling flecks of silver and gold, the spellbinding colours of its skin. Is this what a basking shark would see if it cruised past? Is this how a seal would stare back?

The tide is turning. I feel it. Luke calls us towards him, leading us 'home' to the boat. The last few metres are tiring and laborious, so strong is the water's pull. But we make it, one by one, and hoist ourselves on to the safety of the deck. After refreshments, we're motoring back to the sound. The shark hunt has resumed.

Three hours of slow cruising later, still no sharks have appeared. Gradually the sky darkens. All these non-existent fins will be even harder to spot. Midway through the afternoon, a growing swell makes Rosie, the girlfriend from the family on our boat, vomit her packed lunch into the surf. The clouds cluster over our heads. We are still in our wetsuits, damp and cooling. I want to take mine off and get warm, but I can't miss my chance to jump into the water.

Breaking an ultra-long silence, Gillian admits that, 'The sharks could be passing half a metre under the boat and we wouldn't see them.' I wonder how many have swept beside us today completely unnoticed. Could be ten. Could be one hundred.

Our third full day on the Isle of Coll is a washout. Again it is raining, the wind too strong for the boats. The disappointed group of three-dayers catch their ferry back to Oban – Kay and Sam included. There will be no sharks for them this trip. There may be no sharks for anyone.

That evening, when the weather becomes more placid, we head out for another short ride, seeing schools of dolphins from the boat, even two brief moments of minke whale. But there is not a single shark. Where once I had bad dreams about swimming with fish, that night I have dreams of not swimming with them at all. Tight knots squeeze my stomach as I watch myself leaving the island without an encounter. For so many nights I have wrestled with the thought of sharing the water with basking sharks. I have spent money, time and energy – so much of it all to see a big fish; to turn around my feelings and my fortunes. But the big fish don't want to see me. Not here. Their purposes and mine don't overlap.

In the morning of our last day in the Hebrides, our group

gathers on the boat for the final time, all too aware of how limited our chances of a shark swim have become. In seven hours we must be back on dry land. We have already spent more than double that on the water with no luck.

Gillian is our only guide today, and unlike Luke she does not rely on binoculars. Nor does she offer us positive titbits. Nothing like her counterpart's *I'm confidents*. Instead she uses words like 'might' and 'could'. Phrases like 'It's possible . . .' and 'You never know.'

We are, again, patrolling Gunna Sound, and coming back to this spot is in no way an uplifting reunion. The most eventful part of the morning is when two swimmers are forced by their bladders to climb overboard and pee. As they do their best to flush through their wetsuits, the rest of us keep our eyes on a coastal outcrop, playing a lazy game of *Rock or Seal?*

There are now less than four hours to go until home-time, with nothing to do but breathe boat fumes, and fish out the odd piece of jettisoned plastic.

During a particularly sleepy lull, Gillian shouts, 'Shark!' and shocks us all. I get to my feet. *It's a false alarm*, I tell myself, urging my pulmonary system to slow down.

'Where?' I say. 'Where is it?'

She points in the direction of a buoy that we've circled countless times over the past few days. I can't see a shark. I can't see it.

No one can see it.

Suddenly: the unmistakable sight of a dorsal fin. Sharp. Shining. Looming large. Moving forward. The skipper swerves the boat around and we fix our eyes on the apex as we approach. The dart of it is pointing into the tide.

'No way,' I say. 'No way.'

Every nerve in my body is taut.

'It can't be real,' I say. 'No way. No way.' My muscles are quivering. It looks awfully big, this dorsal fin. Awfully like it belongs to a very big shark.

'There's the tailfin,' shouts Gillian. 'It's a large one. Must be about 6 metres long.' *Six metres*, I think. *Six metres.* My mouth is dry but I swallow regardless.

We are so close to the fish now I could stick my face under the water and be seeing it; see that whole 6 metres in its entirety.

'Are we going to swim?' I ask Gillian.

She does not answer. Nobody answers. I want to know what to do. This is what I've been waiting for. I want to know why nothing's happening. Should I jump?

'It's feeding,' calls the skipper, staring down from where he stands. And I think I see, I'm sure I see, a rippling patch of white beneath the surface. That would be its gaping mouth. Its vast, bony interior. *Do I want to swim?* I ask myself. *Do I want to get in?*

'It's heading for the boat!' shouts Rosie. And she's right. The dorsal fin is heading towards us.

It's a plankton eater. It doesn't eat boats. It doesn't eat people. People are worse than sharks. People are worse than sharks.

There's a glimpse of darkness. Another white flash. The fin shrinks. The shark is sinking down to pass underneath us. We race to the other side of the deck. The fin does not come back up.

'Keep watching,' says Gillian.

And we do. We keep watching the waves.

16

Breath Hold

'You reach for your buddy and . . . you miss. What happened?'

ADAPTING TO THE UNDERWATER WORLD,
PADI OPEN WATER MANUAL, 1999–2007

A long ferry ride to the mainland. A long train ride to London. A long tube ride to home, where Max waits to greet me with a consolatory hug. While he starts to cook, I unpack my bag, then head to the bathroom to sit on the cool toilet lid. There's a poster on the back of my bathroom door, a diagram of the ocean. It names the layers of the sea. Illustrates some of the creatures you might find in each of the zones. I've been using it as a tool to help me better desensitise to them. In the highest layer, the photic layer, yet plainly out of sight of the scuba diver, a basking shark is swimming with its mouth open. I study its form, so much larger than the human's. I'm struck again, as if for the first time, that nowhere on this poster swims a whale shark.

Max knocks on the door. 'Can I come in?'

'Mm.'

He enters smelling of fried onions and spices, and perches beside the sink. 'I'm sorry you're feeling sad,' he says. 'Onwards and upwards?'

'Maybe,' I say. 'Maybe not.'

I am dimly aware of him waiting for me to elaborate. But what can I say, except voice the same concerns. *I've missed out again. I don't know why I keep going. I wish I could give up the fish, but I can't.* Beneath all that, however, lie deeper worries. Whirlpools. Unspoken statements. *Maybe this misplaced attention is why I lost Ted.* And: *Maybe it stopped me from saving Granny.* And: *Maybe it's going to kill our relationship too.* By the time I look back up, these thoughts are tangled like fishing wire in my mouth, and Max has slipped away, shutting the bathroom door behind him.

There are three months between my Hebrides trip and my journey to Mafia Island. That's three months to pick myself up again, to do everything I need to do to before I set out for what must be, what surely has to be, my final bid for giant sharks. I'm not a marine biologist like Simon Pierce. I cannot continue to focus on fish for ever.

The time keeps rolling forward. Seeing only darkness on the horizon, fighting the urge to drop everything and Canute myself against it, I lumber on with my day-to-day activities. I write for money, I meditate, I write to keep busy, I swim, I grip the floor tiles in the pool and do my best to expand my lungs. As I gradually tick the imperatives off my list (the vaccinations, the insurance, the currency, the anti-malarial medication), I have the sensation of constantly holding my breath. My insides are flaring. In one moment I contemplate my approach towards this massive blank patch of Unknown. In the next I order myself to *Stop thinking like that. They are fish. They are not The Unknown.* I can hardly bear to acknowledge that what comes after the fish will be worse. That then I will be facing The Real Unknown.

Occasionally new diving contacts – friends of friends of friends – still get in touch, and I seize upon whatever last pieces of advice they can give me. One of them is Jamie Hull, an ex-policeman, ex-army reservist, who, like my ex-RAF contact Rob, teaches diving to aid recovery in the Help for Heroes scuba diving programme. If talking to Jamie won't help build perspective, I suspect that nothing can.

In 2007 in Florida, while training independently to achieve his pilot's licence, Jamie was involved in a horrific, life-changing accident. The engine of the plane he was flying caught fire in mid-air, and his body burned in the cockpit as he attempted to make an emergency landing.

'On a level of one to ten, the pain was like a perfect ten,' he tells me. 'I didn't think it was even possible to experience pain at that kind of level, and that alone put me into a deep chronic shock almost immediately. I mustered every ounce of strength just holding on.' He believes that rescuers must have reached him very quickly after he jumped, still on fire, from the wing of the plane, mere moments before he crash-landed. But, even then, 'the doctors didn't believe I was going to make it – there was about a 5 per cent chance of survival.'

In order to treat his injuries, these doctors put Jamie into a drug-induced coma that lasted six months. He remembers nothing of it. Following that he battled all sorts of complications. Kidney shutdown, pneumonia, septicaemia, 'pretty much every infection under the sun.' After two solid years in hospital, Jamie was discharged. Four years after his accident, in the midst of a six-year period of surgeries, his former PADI teacher invited him to Egypt for a break – to dive again. All of his expenses would be covered. Not without hesitation, Jamie accepted.

It's hard to imagine how nervous that impending prospect must have made him. Jamie, already so vulnerable, was preparing to enter yet another high-risk environment, about to zip up a wetsuit over his badly damaged skin, endeavouring to mend himself in shark-infested waters. He knew that it would be scary: 'there was always some element of fear or trepidation in scuba diving for me.' But still he went along. And took that giant stride off the back of the boat.

'It took a lot of courage,' he says, 'being gravely injured . . . but to my surprise – to my astonishment – diving helped me in more ways than one.' The activity built up his self-esteem, he says. Moving against the resistance of the ocean had physical benefits. Plus the saltwater itself seemed to markedly speed up his skin's healing process.

'It's like rehab magnified,' he says. 'I'll always be a wounded chap, but I'm turning the negative into a positive.'

Jamie tells me he stills feels fear in the ocean. He can understand why other people might feel fear in the ocean too. But now he helps them progress through the medium of water, using their training to give himself focus. In fact, he is travelling to Koh Tao the day after we speak, where he'll train to become a PADI course director – a professional rank widely recognised as the highest in recreational diving.

As Jamie puts it, 'Bad things can happen in life if you choose to get off the sofa and do stuff.' That's the risk we all have to take: the risk of being alive. And staying alive.

After our call is over, admiring Jamie's ability to accept an uncertain future, I sink into the mattress, stare out of the window, and think about Koh Tao. The thought of Jamie travelling there tomorrow takes me back. To my flustered night-time arrival at the hostel. To my awkward pool practice with Terry. To my first dives in open water. All of it feels so long ago.

Since then I've swum with so many fish and met so many people. I've spoken with a record-breaking adventurer. With a committed corpse retriever. With a bathynaut. With a merman. My focus has mushroomed from fish to fear, via shipwrecks, drownings, a Shropshire shed, underwater caves and hospital chambers. Now my next stop, my final stop, will be Mafia Island. But in spite of everything I've learned – or, perhaps, because of it – I still can't be sure of achieving a positive outcome.

'You never know what's around the next corner,' said Jamie. Which must be the only knowable thing there is.

Part Three

We Swim

17

Mafiosa

'Okay, this is it! You're about to go under.'

BREATHING UNDERWATER,
PADI OPEN WATER MANUAL, 1999–2007

It's the morning of my flight to Tanzania. Max wakes up beside me, and wraps his bed-warm arms around my waist.

'How did you sleep?' he asks.

'Amazingly well,' I say, 'all things considered.'

'Today's the day.'

'Yep.'

He tightens his grip. 'How are you feeling?'

I think about this for a moment. I turn to him. 'Like I'm going to die.'

'You say that all the time,' he sighs. His grip gets tighter. 'Don't die.'

'Maybe I'm OK with dying. I need to be OK with it.'

'OK ...'

'I mean, it's going to happen sometime, right? It might not be swimming with whale sharks that gets me.'

'I'm telling you, Georgie, it won't be.'

'Right. I might be hit by a bus on my way to Heathrow. Or fall from the sky over Dar es Salaam. Or miss one of my flights and succumb to a stress-induced heart attack.'

Max pauses. 'It's possible.'

Both of us are quiet for a moment. 'I don't *want* to die on this trip,' I say.

'Good.'

'But I think that I probably will.'

'Oh.'

'It was genuinely excellent knowing you, Max.'

'It was excellent knowing you too.'

Then I cry.

Max leaves after we've sketched out my funeral plans (cardboard coffin, pasta-bake wake, final resting place with Granny Codd). I'm convinced I'll never see him again, and that makes me cry a second time. Then a third. This is getting ridiculous. I have places to be.

Several hours later, at Heathrow, the first portent of my journey shows itself. As I try very hard to anchor myself in the moment, I glance up at the ceiling over my seat in Terminal 4. The whole hall has been decorated with long, slightly curved white strips of wood or plastic, producing an effect that's like the rib bones of a fish. I'm inside the belly of the whale shark, and haven't even taken off from London.

At risk of being carried away by my nerves, I try reaching again for stability. My mind eventually settles on the four components of the Anxiety Equation.

First, likelihood. What's the likelihood of being attacked and eaten by a whale shark? Non-existent, according to Simon. Even if one mistook me for a school of krill (unlikely), their throats are the size of an apple. *The size of an apple.* I consider picking the phrase for my new mantra.

Second, awfulness. How awful would it be if a whale

shark attacked and ate me? That is a tough one to answer. I'm certain it would be bad – being eaten alive by anything can't be fun. But by pushing myself I can think of worse fates to encounter. Feeling my blood bubble like Pepsi-Cola. Convulsing at the bottom of the Blue Hole. Being turned inside-out by a diving bell. Watching Mum or Max being swallowed instead. All of those options are off the cards, and that thought brings me relief.

Third, rescue. Who will be there to support me when I look for whale sharks? I can answer this more easily: Simon and his colleague, Chris. I've paid extra to stay in the same lodge as both of them, to pitch for the role of sidekick during their giant-fish-finding antics. What's more, on Simon's advice, I've also arranged to meet up with a very important islander on my first day: the impressively named Liberatus, or Libber, the skipper who first brought the concept of whale shark tourism to Mafia. Before Simon and Chris can wrap up the guided holiday they're running, I'll be able to start my shark search on one of Libber's boats. Also on that boat will be other shark-seekers. Other shark-seekers like me. Never mind that they don't know me. Never mind that they may be inclined to abandon me quickly when they do. Whale sharks will have brought us together. These people can be my rescuers.

Lastly, the final element of the equation: ability to cope. How should I expect to deal with the whale shark? CBT therapist Emma told me this step involved thinking back to traumatic events. On my hard-backed chair in departures, grounded by the sight of families shopping, by bags of duty-free, by announcements for late passengers and delayed planes, I let the memories come. My first panic attack at the Great Barrier Reef. Goldfish dying around me in Mum's back garden. Faceless dolphins circling my legs. Ted's pained expression as he left. Being pulled out by my feet from a freezing lake. Coming back into the room to see Granny Codd's body. Carrying on without her. I don't know if I can say I've coped but I've tried. And I'm still here. Still able to try. Perhaps that's coping. Kind of. In a way.

Seventeen hours later, having stopped over in Nairobi and Dar es Salaam, I'm embarking on the final leg of my journey, buckled into a tiny plane for Mafia. Our flight time, says the co-pilot, turning to face us ('us' being a grand total of eight passengers), will be somewhere in the region of thirty-five minutes.

As the wheels leave the tarmac, I feel like I leave my own body. Some other Georgie must be in Tanzania – a part of the world I've never seen before – investing in this last-gasp attempt to see whale sharks. Why on earth would *I* be on a rattling plane in pursuit of enormous fish, trying to use the experience to become a better person? That would be absurd.

But both Georgies unite as we look out of the window, crossing the western edge of the Indian Ocean. Both of us see the same thing in the skies surrounding us: bulbous whale sharks made from vapour; cloud-creatures the size of aircraft carriers floating on the breeze. Beneath them lies an eternity of turquoise, shadows of clouds casting doubts. Occasionally there are ripples, cracks in the ocean. Some of these cracks could be whale sharks. I want to know which ones. But no matter how hard I press my face against the glass the results are inconclusive.

Soon we are approaching a palm-cropped island. Not a small patch of sand but a fully grown, real-world, inhabited destination. Roughly 30 miles long by 9 across, it stretches further than I can see from my buckled position. The section in my eyeline is flat and green, stitched together with brown roads, dry clearings, and a small-town cluster of one-storey dwellings. The plane descends to a concrete strip. Our wheels drop to meet it gently. The propeller slows. The co-pilot turns to face us once again.

'Welcome to Mafia,' he says. I applaud.

Grabbing my rucksack from the hold, I follow my fellow passengers into the island's pint-sized terminal building. Five steps later I'm out of it already. A local man turns to greet me.

'Georgie?' he asks. 'Georgie Code?'

'Almost.'

He leads me to an autorickshaw, my last mode of transportation for the day. Seamless. Just as carefully plotted arrivals should always be.

I've read that Mafia Island's name is likely to have come from the Arabic word *morfiyeh*, meaning 'group' or 'archipelago'. Alternatively it may have been derived from a phrase in Swahili meaning 'healthy dwelling place.' Despite my own positive introduction to Mafia, I can't help but consider the name in terms of its Sicilian connotations: gangsters with 'swagger' or 'boldness'. I think of severed horse heads in beds. Pacts going terribly wrong. In truth, so far, any evidence of sinister undertones here is sparse. While there are signs of animals in the thatch-covered bedroom I'll be sleeping in, none are of the decapitated variety. All sound very much alive, especially the wild rats that scamper, squeaking, from one side of the roof to the other. The occasional gecko climbs the wall in hot pursuit of the nearest ant or fly.

While there's still a sun up to light my way, I venture out to find the nearest place to eat, guided by one of the helpers at my lodge, an old man who doesn't speak English. En route, my unshakeable tourist-ness attracts multiple greetings – various *Jambo*s and *Mambo*s – as well as stares all round. I start to suspect this is not a side of the island that sees many outsiders, a hunch that's further strengthened when a group of schoolchildren wrapped in long skirts runs up to us.

'Mambo! Mambo! Hello! English! Where are you from?'

As I answer, one boy takes my hand. Another, while I'm distracted, pulls my hair. It seems he wants to know what the straight strands feel like between his fingers, and he doesn't pull hard or maliciously. Still, the action surprises me; when I say 'Hey!' the group legs it, giggling off down the track.

I'm escorted to a one-room hut with a gas stove out the front, and left there to be served a plate of cold rice and beans, along with a glass of sweet juice made from pineapple and cardamom. I devour it all, my first meal since 4 a.m., thirteen hours earlier, and tell my stomach that it must not, under any circumstances, contract any sort of food poisoning. Cold rice, though ... Flies wading through my plate ... I fear I'm asking too much.

When I get back to the lodge there is still no one around. No hostel vibes or people to distract me. Simon is staying elsewhere for the next two nights, and Chris is presumably still out with their fund-generating group of holidaymakers. I hope he comes back. I hope both of them do. Already I'm feeling lonely. I try to send a message to Max but the internet won't work. I put my phone away, sit on a chair in a lounge-type space which is open to the elements, and look out over the flat-calm sea below. Sailboats slide through the gaps between palm trees. Insects trill like steam kettles boiling over. This time of year in Mafia, said Simon, is peak whale shark season. According to him, whale shark sightings at this time are effectively *guaranteed*.

Today I've seen a man in a whale shark T-shirt, a statue of a whale shark outside the airport, even a whale shark mural at the entrance of my lodge. In theory, if my stomach stays strong, I'll soon be seeing more than mere representations. The whale sharks I'll see will be real and large, barrelling through the water. At that point all of my searching will be over.

I hear a monkey shriek with distress in the foliage.

'That's right,' I say. 'I feel you.'

Overnight, during a shallow, jet-lagged sleep, the beats of a nearby disco trick my brain. For almost an hour I'm convinced that Chris, a man I've never met, has arranged a show of music for my arrival; that every single song he plays is a special Swahili number about whale sharks.

'Thank you,' I murmur. 'Maybe just one more – then I really must go to sleep.'

In the morning, still disorientated, I stagger out of the room and up to the al fresco dining area. I'm hoping I'm not too late to find breakfast. There I spot a man who looks like the various pictures I've seen of Chris.

It is Chris.

'Welcome!' he says as I approach, breaking off from a small plate of pancakes to shake my hand. 'Are you Georgie?'

'Thank goodness,' I say. 'You're here!'

Chris is a Swiss-born ecologist, and was Simon's first PhD student, pursuing the study of whale sharks with an Australian university. Now in full possession of his doctorate, he continues his whale shark research as the Marine Megafauna Foundation's principal scientist. At his request, I pull up a chair and within minutes I learn that his partner makes her living as a specialist on plankton.

'Match made in heaven,' I say.

'Indeed,' Chris says with a grin.

A cheerful girl from the lodge pads over to our table with

a plate of fresh fruit, and already I feel so much more at ease than I predicted for my first full day on the island. Until, that is, I ask the fatal question.

'So ... have you seen many whale sharks since you got here?'

Chris is chewing pancake. 'Mm.'

I wait for him to clear his mouth, expecting to hear an answer like ten a day. Possibly twenty.

Then Chris shakes his head. Swallows. 'Not so many.'

Of course they haven't. Of *course*.

'The winds this year aren't doing what they should,' he explains. 'Normally they push the plankton this way – to Mafia – then the whale sharks come up to eat. But that hasn't happened. For some reason, we're not sure, it's late.' Chris tells me that where they'd normally see multiple whale sharks a day, on the trip that he and Simon are currently running they've been finding it hard to spot even one. 'Most of the whale sharks we see here live in this area all year round,' he says. 'But they're mostly offshore. And of course they are much harder to find when they're not feeding at the surface.'

So many miles travelled, so much more money spent, only, again, to meet with bad luck. I stab at a piece of mango. Count to ten.

Chris gestures to the horizon. 'In other years we've seen them feeding even from where we're sitting – you can watch them while you eat.'

'Not this year.'

He shakes his head again. 'Not yet. You're here for a few days though, aren't you? Going out with one of Libber's boats tomorrow?'

I nod. Spear a banana.

'And I hear you might be coming out with me and Simon at the start of next week?'

'If you'll have me,' I say, more hopefully. 'If there's space.'

'I'm sure there'll be space,' Chris says. He leans back in his chair, a picture of calm. 'Don't worry,' he says. 'You're going to find your whale shark.'

After Chris leaves for his day at sea, I head to the nearest strip of shore to road-test my snorkel and mask. Dense clumps of palm trees and mangroves trap and pass the heat between them. The sandy-floored chamber their branches create is quiet. Eerily so. At the nearest wide gap between the roots I step into the shallows. The tide is ebbing. In an hour, there'll be no water left. I kneel on the sea floor, peek through my mask, and push myself off, making a starfish shape with my arms and legs. At breakfast, Chris told me jellyfish floated here, but that they wouldn't hurt me one bit. Sure enough, within moments, a brown orb the size of a tennis ball bobs into my field of vision. I recoil and veer away – straight towards another. These jellies are frilly and speckled, with ominous-looking tentacles. *They're harmless,* I say to myself. Another one appears in my line of sight. *They're coming for me.* I yelp and jump out to safety.

Rinsed and dressed, I try to restore my bruised confidence with a solo trek along the beach to town. Only, in this activity, too, I feel exposed. The locals are going about their daily business, comfortable, smiling, buying their supplies. But many of them are also staring at me. Children dare each other to shout 'Mambo!' A man on a scooter beeps and says hello. Two women sit and whisper, eyeing up my plain T-shirt and trousers, then jointly burst out laughing. I wish Max was here. On my own, I'm the only tourist. I feel so out of place.

Buying a portion of chips with broken Swahili – then finding, to my dismay, that they're not only cold but stale – I scuttle back to the beach, where fishermen stop what they're doing to watch me pass. From the top of a tall wooden post, a crow hangs upside-down in a loop of wire that has been tightly wound around its stick-like legs. The bird wasn't there ten minutes ago, I'm sure. It looks like a fresh kill.

I pick up the pace, agitated. For the rest of the day, I hide in the lodge and half-read, half-gape at the sea, trying to tell myself that I've overreacted; that, contrary to my instincts, the islanders aren't conspiring for my demise. I know they've got better things to do with their lives. I know I need to stop being paranoid. Even so, I'm greatly relieved when I hear a familiar voice in the compound – a voice with a New Zealand lilt. It is Simon, come to drop off Chris and say hello before his last night with their tour group.

'How's it going?' he asks me.

'Nice!' I say, with an overloud enthusiasm. 'The island's . . . very beautiful!'

'Busy day?'

'I, uh, went into town! Saw a dead crow hanging from a pole! Oh, and some creepy jellyfish followed me this morning!'

'Good sign,' says Chris. 'We want you attracting the fish.'

I cock my head. I hadn't thought of that.

Simon explains their plans for the next few days: that tomorrow, during my first boat ride out, they'll be taking their last shark-seeking trip with their group. That the following day, a Sunday, the two of them will stay on land, catching up with their work. Afterwards, on Monday, he and Chris will go out researching. 'You can come with us then,' he says.

'I'd love that,' I say, instantly buzzing at the prospect of their company. 'Thank you so *much*.'

Then Libber appears, their lean and savvy skipper, and I greet him with a smile, buzzing still. Libber knows Mafia's whale sharks better than any islander out here. Arguably, if it wasn't for Libber, neither Simon, nor Chris, nor I would be here right now. I ask if he'll sit, drink a beer, and share his story. He pulls up a chair while twilight falls. Flying foxes flap towards the trees. Simon heads back to his guests.

'I'm a tribesman, a bushman, a hunter,' Libber tells me. 'I grow up on the mainland and I like to see those big animals: rhino, elephant, buffalo. I don't worry. Very interested.' He tells me his brother came out to this island to earn a living from fishing, then encouraged Libber to follow. 'Before, I do not swim,' Libber says. He did not know how to fish either. Or even use a boat. But he became a fisherman all the same, and, when he saw his first whale sharks in the water, his fascination with the creatures ballooned.

'I try to make a research of the whale sharks for four years,' he tells me. 'Try to advertise to the hoteliers. But they were interested only in dugongs [a sea-grass-grazing marine mammal] and sea turtles' – both species that typically reside on the other side of Mafia, within the protected setting of a marine park. 'Nobody is interested in the whale sharks first time,' Libber says. It can't have helped that, although he was trying to promote himself as a shark spotter, he was severely cash-strapped. 'Don't have a boat, don't have an engine, just have an idea.'

The breakthrough came when an American tourist saw whale sharks from his plane over Mafia's waters. He'd been searching for those fish for years, he told his hotelier, and wanted to know if any locals could take him out on the water to see them up-close. It was all systems go for Libber.

'I hired a boat from my friends,' he says. 'I hired petrol. I have no capital.' He took the man under his wing and together they saw 'many whale sharks'. The money Libber earned that day enabled him to make a proper start. His business grew. Then, when Libber invited a US student to research from his boat for free, the resulting report attracted global scientific interest in the island. It was in the wake of that interest that he teamed up with Chris and Simon.

During several years of fine-tuning his own knowledge, Libber has taught many other Mafians to look for the whale sharks. Some of them have now started rival businesses, but Libber does not seem to mind. On the contrary: it all feeds into his plan to crown Mafia Island *The Home of the Whale Shark*.

'Whale shark is my friend,' says Libber. 'One of the family. We have a relationship. They follow me. We meet together. They come to say hello to me.' Libber says he gets a feeling in his gut about where they are. 'They don't let me down,' he says. 'Every day we go and find the whale sharks.'

It sounds like a blissful pairing of man and beast, and I don't want to burst the bubble, but I also want to understand my chances; to set my expectations at the right level.

'I hear the plankton aren't here now,' I say. 'That the whale sharks aren't coming up yet like they should. Is that true?'

For a moment Libber's glow flickers. 'Yes,' he says. 'Until December the northern winds blow' – northern wind being what we, and the whale sharks, are missing.

'So it's possible I won't see them while I'm here?'

Sincerely, solemnly, Libber looks me in the eye, and says, 'You will see the whale sharks.'

'I will?'

'I promise.'

Libber's promise clings to me all night. That's it. My fate in Mafia is apparently sealed. It's just a matter of timing; of when I will see my whale shark. Will it be on the boat with Simon and Chris in two days? Or could it be as soon as tomorrow, when I'm picked up from the shore? I toss around in the bedsheets, overheating. Whenever I shut my eyes sharks drift towards me. Silent. Mouths gaping. I know I need to wait long enough to see those black mouths close. To watch those formidable whale sharks pass me by.

Before leaving, after he finished his beer, Libber assured me a boat would come to take me to the whale sharks at 8 a.m. At 7.15, I sit with my breakfast, very much on edge. In contrast, the sea before me could not be more tranquil. Each boat leaves a mark on its surface like a snail trail. One of those trails will be from Libber's boat; the one I heard come for Chris. I wonder how many whale sharks Libber has led them to already. Perhaps none. I hope it's none.

By 8.47 there's still no boat for me. The owner of my lodge, Carlos, makes a call to Libber's company on my behalf. He is told my skipper is still waiting for passengers. I watch a small team of fisherman unfurl a net, then slink into the water to monitor their catch. The scene prompts me to ask Carlos if he's ever eaten whale shark.

'No, no,' he says with conviction.

'How about the other islanders? Have they eaten it?'

He shakes his head again. 'They're too big,' he says. 'Also,' he adds more quietly, 'the meat is not so good.'

8.54. Still nothing. Not even the sound of an engine. Carlos pauses his morning tasks to make an assessment of the gathering clouds.

'The whale sharks don't like this weather,' he tells me. 'They go . . . ' He holds his hand in front of him and slides it, fingers first, towards the floor. *Down.*

9.01. No boat yet and a wind has just picked up. It's not a northerly. I've watched two boats leave the pier in the last five minutes. Neither is coming this way.

9.05. A third boat has left. Looks like it's heading over.

9.07. Or maybe not. It's going so slowly.

I can't all stand this waiting. I've been to the loo three times in fifteen minutes.

9.08. The sound of the third boat's engine is growing louder. If this is my boat it's going to take us several hours to get anywhere.

9.10. It's coming this way. It's my boat.

Oh God, it's my boat.

Thanking Carlos for his company, I run down the steps to the beach with my fins, mask and snorkel tucked under my arm. Minutes later, I'm wading towards a puttering wooden boat. Above it is a cloth canopy, on which is painted, in black and white, an elongated whale shark. I am invited aboard, and as soon as I swing myself up the vessel sets off again. There are eight people on the boat with me: our guide, Kassim, and his skipper; a group of four blokes from South Africa; a French woman called Delphine, and a Dutch traveller on his fourth gap year, named Marin.

Marin: marine.

Delphine: dolphin.

Codd: fish.

It seems too good to be true.

'Have any of you got fishy names?' I ask the four South Africans.

'Nah,' says the nearest, indicating himself. 'I'm Marcus.' He nods at his two friends opposite. 'That's Bushman Junior and Bushman Senior.'

'Bushman?'

'B-O-E-S-M-A-N,' spells Marcus. 'And this,' he says, pointing next to him, 'is Dieter. So not fishy at all. But we did come to Mafia Island to *go* fishing. Does that count?'

'Not that we've caught anything,' Dieter adds.

'Maybe with a Dolphin and a Marine we have the credentials we need to find a whale shark,' I suggest.

Delphine whoops. 'Yeah! Whale *shark!*' It turns out she has been looking for whale sharks for over twenty years. 'I saw one from the plane when I was coming into Mafia,' she enthuses. 'So *beautiful!*'

'I swam with some a few days ago!' says Marin, flushed with excitement. 'It was *amazing*. So cool! They're so *big*. They came so *close*! I can't wait to do it again.'

Delphine squeals. 'That's so *cool!*'

'Are none of you frightened?' I ask.

A chorus of nopes and shaking heads comes back to me. Fearless, happy, enthusiastic – it strikes me that I've landed exactly the right crew for the morning. Their high spirits buoy me up. Surely there can be nothing to fear when nobody else is worried.

Within half an hour, we're approaching a group of other canopied boats. Kassim suggests that they might have stopped next to a whale shark, and my heartbeat immediately booms. Marin grabs his mask and snorkel, starts shuffling into his fins.

'There's no time to prepare otherwise,' he confides. 'When the shark's there it's just *go, go, go!*'

My face drops. I'm not ready for this. But I root around for my own equipment anyway. Delphine is whooping again. The four South Africans banter with each other, a hearty exchange of Afrikaans that has them all splitting their sides. The scene seems surreal. This is not how I expected things to be before meeting a whale shark. I expected tension, reverence, some acknowledgement of the power of life and the ocean. A cargo of nerves. But my fellow boat people just aren't into that.

We get to within 50 metres of the other tourist vessels. Kassim calls across to another guide and skipper. The guide shouts back. Their conversation goes on for a minute or more. Marin is standing, poised, ready to dive. Delphin is adjusting her fins. I am staring into the water beside us. *Is that it? Or is it a shadow?* Even the South Africans have gone quiet. Then Kassim addresses our skipper, who revs the engine. We start to pull away.

'Are we going in?' asks Marcus.

'No whale shark,' Kassim says.

Before stopping to consider the implications of what I'm about to say, I apologise to the group.

'My fault,' I announce. 'Any time I look for the big things they don't show up. I mean, I've seen one spotted eagle ray in about three years. But to be honest I wasn't really any-where near it.'

Marcus stares at me. 'So if we don't see anything today, it's because of you?'

I shrug, already feeling a twinge of regret. 'Possibly.'

I may be imagining things, but over the next twenty minutes it seems like the spirits of the group start to dip. An hour after that it's clear: I'm not imagining things. Conversations have more or less ground to a halt. In place of whooping, Delphine is lighting cigarette after cigarette. Kassim stands on the prow staring into the water. Marin waits next to him, silent.

'Go and sit on that buoy, Georgie,' says Marcus, as we circle the only landmark out here once again. 'We don't want your curse on our boat any more.'

'I don't want it either,' I say, mopily. Then something occurs to me, a memory of a phrase. Perhaps I'm not the only one to blame. 'Didn't you say you guys hadn't caught anything when you were fishing?' I ask.

'That's probably your fault too,' Marcus snaps back. Dieter and the Bushmen chuckle.

Kassim interrupts us with a shout. 'Dolphins!'

We all stand to look.

'Let's go in,' says Marcus.

'Yes!' shouts Delphine.

Marin springs over to his mask and snorkel.

'Is swimming with dolphins allowed?' I ask. 'It's not allowed in England.'

'You're not in England now,' says Bushman Junior.

Kassim seems reluctant to let us go in. 'They'll swim away,' he tells us. 'Very fast. Quick.'

'But we're not seeing any whale sharks,' says Marcus. 'Might as well see something.' He grabs his fins. 'Let's go,' he says to his friends.

I watch a fin rise and fall. 'Is it allowed?' I ask Kassim.

He shrugs. 'If you want.'

'We can go?' asks Marin. 'Can we go?'

Kassim nods. Marin jumps in. Afraid of missing out, I jump in behind him. The others follow but I'm not looking at them. The sea floor is about 10 metres down, and speckled with starfish. Twenty meters away is an adult dolphin with a young calf. That's where I'm looking. The adult is watching me and Marin. It starts to come closer. Then it changes its mind and ushers its calf away, escaping into the blue.

No more dolphins.

I peer around me regardless. Maybe this is the time for a whale shark to come. I whisper into my snorkel: 'Let me move on. Just appear and let me move on.'

But no whale shark appears.

One by one we drag ourselves on to our boat, flopping into a mess of sandals and backpacks. The motoring continues. Kassim cuts up a watermelon, passing out the pieces. Delphine starts to whistle.

'Here, whale shark,' she calls.

I stare harder than ever into the crystal water. Everything under the surface looks like a whale shark, but nothing looks enough like a whale shark to be one.

The sky clears. The wind dies down. We have been on the boat for about three hours, with only shards of watermelon pips in our teeth to show for all that waiting.

'It was about this time the other day when we saw them,' says Marin. He is clearly clutching at straws, but the statement gives me hope. It has to. Otherwise I only feel the burden of bad luck.

Getting more impatient, Marcus asks Kassim why he doesn't wear sunglasses while looking for the sharks. 'You'd see more with good sunglasses,' he says.

Kassim doesn't understand.

'Take mine,' says Marcus. 'Take these.' He passes them up.

Kassim puts them on and resumes his watch over the water. Perhaps Marcus's lenses will make a difference. Perhaps not. Ten minutes later still nothing has changed.

'Let me clean them,' Marcus says. He takes them back and polishes them with a tissue. 'Here,' he says. 'Try that.'

All of us are slumped against the inside of the boat. All except Kassim, who's alert on the prow, throwing the occasional thumbs up back to Marcus.

Half an hour later, Kassim turns around again.

'Whale shark,' he says with certainty, pointing into the water. 'Whale shark. There.'

18

To the Shark

'If you see a shark . . . remain still and calm . . . Watch it
and see what it does. Chances are it's just passing through.
And enjoy.'

AQUATIC ANIMALS,
PADI OPEN WATER MANUAL, 1999–2007

'Whale shark,' Kassim repeats. He talks to the skipper.
Instructs him in Swahili. Gestures as to where to
manoeuvre the boat.

I have no time. I'm not prepared. Delphine and Marin
are squealing with pleasure, throwing on their kit. I pick up
my fins. I pick up my mask and snorkel. *This isn't real*, I tell
myself. *It isn't happening.* But the skipper is getting us into
position regardless. There is so much movement, a volume
of activity too great for this small space. My brain feels like
it's being ambushed by a whirlwind.

Marin takes his place on the prow, all good to go, then
sees me fretting, trying and failing to work out what to do
next. He wriggles along. Makes a space next to him and
pats it. Overwhelmed, I thank him and clunk my limbs

into position beside him. Yes. This is what I'm supposed to be doing.

The water pulls at the tips of my fins. I can't see the whale shark, but Kassim is still pointing down.

'Is it there?' I ask.

'Yes,' says Kassim, delighted. 'Go, go, go!'

I hesitate.

Marin leaps in.

'Go, go, go, go, go!'

My muscles respond where my mind cannot. I throw myself into the water face down. As the bubbles clear my mask is filled with whale shark. A real, live, actual whale shark. I shriek into my snorkel. It's about 15 metres below me, swimming forward, from my left to my right, and it looks huge. Completely huge. *Not real*, my mind transmits to me, *Not real*. I cannot compute what I'm seeing. *Not real. Not real. Not real.* As if the scene before me wasn't outlandish enough, there are also two slender, shark-like fish swimming with the whale shark, each one as long as a person. They peel away from the whale shark and approach Delphine. These are cobia, or kingfish, I learn later, and they look like minions to a giant overlord, startling me with the fierceness of their gaze – though they're nowhere near as startling as the spotted titan they guard.

The whale shark glides at a speed I'm not sure I can keep pace with. Jolted into action, I start to swim. I want to be near the whale shark. Not 15 or 20 metres away but up close. I want to see it next to me. Its powerful tail. Its dots and lines. Its eyes. Its massive mouth. I want to feel like the tiniest thing in the world.

But I'm not fast enough.

I hear the sound of an engine and look up. Kassim is beckoning me in.

'Come, come. We take you closer.'

I heave myself aboard. The others follow.

'I can get a new tattoo!' Delphine cheers. 'A whale shark, right on my leg!'

'Amazing!' says Marin. 'They're so amazing!'

The boat's motor revs.

'Go, go, go, go, go!' says Kassim.

We jump off a second time, slightly closer. And even though I now have a better idea of what to expect, the sight of a whale shark beneath me is still unbelievably shocking. I squeal again into my snorkel, '*Eeeeeeeeeeee*', producing the noise as automatically as the quick, heavy breaths I'm taking. Meanwhile the shark remains at about 15 metres down. It is swimming beautifully, swaying like the pendulum of a masterfully crafted clock. Despite all the prep talks I've given myself since the Hebrides – that the whale shark is a fish and not a concept – the sight seems hypnotic; a symbol created to draw me out of my mind. I am duly spellbound, but kick along with it as hard as I can, telling myself *This is happening, actually happening*, but not being able to make the connection; not feeling it as real.

When Marin dives to get closer, my herd instincts kick in and I dive too, desperate to see the shark for myself, to genuinely see it – stare into those eyes, that mouth – but the nearer I get and the larger it grows, the more I realise: I'm still unprepared. In fact I have dived too far for the breath in my lungs. I look up. The surface of the sea is suddenly very far away. Panicking, I rush towards the air, feeling like a total fool, regretting my decision not to practise with the freedivers when I had the opportunity.

I catch my breath at the surface, inhaling great gulps, and become aware of more engine noises around me. All the other tourist boats in the area are coming. All these tourists have paid for their trips and all want to see their whale shark. I scramble onboard our own boat. Others follow. Everyone except wiry Marin, who is still in the water, still chasing the shark. Our skipper takes the rest of us forward again. Then 'Go, go, go!' says Kassim.

This time as I try to follow the whale shark, the sea starts filling with people, strangers coming from nowhere. They are splashing like crazy. I wonder if I look crazy too. I swim through a gap between two of them, trying to hold my focus, willing the whale shark to come up to me, to ignore all the noise in the water. I urge it to sense me, to choose me, to test me, to recognise how much it means to me, even though I know that's impossible. Moments later the shark does rise a little, and I see the shape of its claspers underneath. This whale shark is a male.

As three, four, five more boats' worth of passengers cascade into the water, the whale shark sinks again. I feel myself tiring. As soon as I stop I completely lose sight of the shark. All I can see is people, thrashing madly. I try to count how many there are but once I get past twenty-five my brain won't focus. More than twenty-five people seems like too much for one shark.

Our boat comes to pick me up. I hitch a lift, then jump back into the water. The shark doesn't come any closer, doesn't rise to the surface, or scare me with its mouth. It just carries on swimming, a touch too deep, indifferent to us all.

I am still in a state of disbelief by the time the evening falls. Simon and Chris are staying out late, so I can't share my experience with them, or make it feel more real. I can't work out if what happened to me was scary. Or brilliant. Or disappointing. I am dazed. One thing I do know: as stupefying as the sight of the whale shark was, it didn't feel like the animal I was waiting for. I wonder if that animal even exists.

Just before I go to bed, Libber sends me a text, apologising for the late pick-up that morning. He writes: 'I want to give offer free of charge tomorrow to go again to see whale shark, do you have time to join with us?'

I don't hesitate to answer. 'Yes,' I write. 'Please.'

I am relived to be going out again, glad to have another chance to see whale sharks, glad to be adopting the official CBT-approved method of *repeat, repeat, repeat*. Even so, stressful visions bed down with me. Behind closed eyes, the whale sharks swim, suspended in the water. I struggle with the thoughts of what I'm hoping for a second time. A closer encounter. Clarity.

My whale shark.

The next morning I'm collected by a fancier boat made from fibreglass. I'm sharing it partly with a local Mafia couple. The woman has apparently never seen whale sharks before. She is dressed as if she's about to go to a fundraiser at the golf club: smart yellow trousers, skin-tight T-shirt, make-up, neatly tied braids. She and her partner sit entwined, absorbed in each other's faces. Also onboard are a British diplomat and his Californian daughter, Charlie and Marley. Both of them saw whale sharks a few days ago, and are keen to chat more about it.

'One of them rose up right next to my wife and I,' says Charlie. 'It was fantastic. *Very* close.'

And that's not it for our band of boaters. Along with Captain Gregory and our spotter, Boniface, is an islander called Shamey (pronounced *sham-ee*), who says that he works as a government rep on Mafia's tourist board.

Shamey is keen to talk. 'This area used to be coral reef,' he tells me, as our boat scuds over the waves. 'All of it was damaged by the fishermen, blown up. It should be protected because of the whale sharks, just like creatures are protected by the marine park on the other side of the island.' Though it's doubtful what protection that really affords. In the very next breath, Shamey tells me that the island's local dugong population – those chubby, herbivorous mammals supposedly defended by the park – appears to have dwindled to nothing this year. 'The researchers did not find one dugong,' he reports with dismay.

Hopefully the whale shark population here will not go the same way, and rising tourist numbers could work in their favour. That said, in spite of the major income stream that shark-spotting has brought to this island, Shamey says that, even today, not all of the locals respect the animals.

'Some of the fishermen poke them,' he says. 'They hit them with sticks. Some of the sharks have only one eye because the fishermen attack them. We also have one shark here with no dorsal fin. It was cut off.'

Other fishermen value the whale shark for the role it can play in leading them to massive shoals of cash-earning fish, like mackerel. Though sometimes the whale sharks are injured when nets are thrown around them to trap the prey they've unwittingly dredged up.

In one line, Shamey sums up the situation: 'The whale sharks are not protected – this needs to change.'

Our boat approaches an outer buoy that's familiar from our shark patrolling yesterday. Two boats have got there before us. I spy splashing in the water. The shape of tourists furiously swimming. I look at Boniface.

'Whale shark?'

He nods.

With fear and excitement – thrilled that today the whale shark has come so quickly – that *this* will be the time I find what I'm looking for – I race to put on my kit and get into position. We circle the crowd of swimmers. A man at the front lifts his head up, sees us, and points down. *There*, his finger tells us. *It's right there.*

'Go! Go! Go!' Boniface shouts, and I jump into the water, staring down. I can't see a thing but blue. I look up. Look around. The local woman jumps in behind me, still wearing her make-up and T-shirt and bright yellow trousers. Is the whale shark underneath her? Where has it gone? I search for the man at the front of the crowd. He is coming closer. Still pointing into the deep. Surely I should be able to see it by now. The man raises his head and then his eyebrows. Points down again. *There.*

I fix my eyes in the water and see what might be a whale shark, or what might be the shadow of a whale shark. Whatever it is it's slowly swaying, perhaps 30 or 40 metres beneath my dangling fins. I try to follow, though I'm unable to even see the shark's patterned white markings – they blend too well with the shafts of light from the surface. Now all I can see is a dark outline in dark water. Again I have the sense of hypnosis, of the whale shark leading me on. Its outline flickers. Is gone. There it is again. And then it has vanished. A trick of the eye. A mirage.

I return to the lodge two hours later, tired and red with sunburn. Chris and Simon are sat at one of the dining tables. With them sits their visiting friend, Rilke, who helped them train whale shark operators on Mafia several years ago. Beside her is her smiling partner, Holly. Their foursome has just finished lunch, and they warmly call me over. I feel like I'm invading – Rilke hasn't seen Simon and Chris for ages; they must have hours of catching up to do – but I'm welcomed straight into the fold.

'Take a seat!' says Simon.

'How did it go?' asks Chris.

Not wanting to spoil the mood with negativity, I try to maintain an upbeat tone as I tell them about my last two days of sightings: how bad luck meant my first boat buddies had threatened to leave me marooned on that buoy; how long it took to find anything; how, when we did, the sharks didn't come close; that the waters were teeming with people.

When I finish Simon says, 'That's not great.' He says the operators are supposed to cap the swimmers at ten. 'But then it's hard to stop tourists throwing themselves in when the shark sightings are down.' He sighs. 'Normally this time of year you'd get much better interactions. The operators would be a little less desperate, a little less pressured to get all their customers in and keep them happy.'

'We'll try to get you closer tomorrow,' says Chris. 'As for the buoy thing, if your buddies *had* left you out there you would have probably seen loads of whale sharks. We get very good activity at that buoy.' He laughs. 'The joke's on them!'

I laugh too. My chest lightens.

A plan for the next day is made: the five of us will leave first thing in the morning and head back to the buoy in question, with Libber himself at the helm. Simon and Chris will be aiming to gather data, taking photos and skin biopsies. They say that Rilke, Holly and I can help out and keep them company.

It all sounds very exciting. I want to celebrate. But part of me is still heavy, and pulling the other parts down. These people have been so friendly to me. I can't bring myself to deceive them. I clear my throat.

'You know I'm cursed, don't you?' I say.

'We do,' says Chris. 'But luckily the whale sharks don't.'

We rise super early, up with the dawn, and sit having breakfast together. On my own last night, I was panicking still, taunting myself with the image of a tick-tocking tail in the water. Now, in friendly company, I'm calm. Rilke tells me about all the times she's been swimming with whale sharks. She tells me how, sometimes, when a single tourist became scared on one of her boats, she could see the others crumbling.

'That fear is infectious,' she says. 'It really spreads.' She refers to a place in Sardinia, where her grandmother used to live. Its residents' fear of the ocean spread so widely there, she says, that the town built its houses to face away from the coast. 'I'm not sure how true this story is though,' she confesses shortly afterwards. 'My grandmother hated that town. She probably made it up just to be mean.'

Fired up by the subject nevertheless, Simon chips in to explain how different nationalities have evolved to express different kinds of panic.

'Americans die more loudly,' he tells us. 'The Japanese do it quietly, so you don't even know they're in trouble until it's too late.' He says the phenomenon is known in certain circles as 'Japanese Shock'. He's even seen it in action on various dives.

'If a whale shark starts to eat me, I'll be screaming,' I assure him. 'Don't you worry.'

Without any conscious thinking, the words I've spoken trigger my panic reflexes. They project imagined pictures to my brain: scream; teeth; swallow; darkness. Privately, bringing to mind what Simon told me about their throats, I try reciting my new mantra to myself — *the size of an apple the size of an apple the size of an apple* — and am chuffed to note that within a couple of minutes I'm more relaxed.

As we finish our pancakes, the sound of Libber's engine fills our ears. Kept steady by the ease of my merry crew, I fetch my things and hurry down to the beach, so eager that I'm first to reach the boat. Libber waves to greet me.

Moments later, the others appear from the treeline.

'To the buoy!' shouts Chris. 'Let's check it out.'

I'm amazed at the effect other people have on my fears, something which seems so obvious when I pause to pay attention. Never mind the waves of uncertainty that have hit me over the past few days, months, years. Sat with a boat of others, positive, confident people who like to chat, who know the whale sharks well and have no cause to be afraid of them, I'm almost entirely serene. Rilke's anecdote about the spread of fear has struck a chord. I realise that, all through this journey, when I've needed to get in the water with something, I've done it because I've been able to take my cues from other people: Terry, teaching me in the Gulf of Thailand; Andrew and Liv in the Andaman; our line of cave divers in Mexico; Marin on my first boat ride to find whale sharks. It's when no one has been available that terror has taken the reins.

I wonder then if the roots of my biggest fears are not based on the great unknown at all. I wonder if they're actually based on loneliness. A fear of experiencing something massive and beyond me – whale sharks, the ocean, death – as a singular being. A mortal being. I think about the dread I had only hours ago, even after all this time and research, even after talking with so many experts about my worries. The dread was all about me being me, completely on my own, confronted by swimming Goliaths.

Perhaps I've not been looking at this phobia in the right way. Perhaps my greatest fear in this project is really the fear of becoming a single 'I', one who can slip through the plates of a whale shark's mouth without being rescued or missed. The fear of not being able to end my own solitude. Of not having friends who'll enter the water with me. Of not being able to choose to say 'we'; *we'll* swim to the shark; we'll swim to the danger *together*.

I couldn't have got this far without the help and advice of others – from Mandi to the Mafians, and everyone else in between. This morning, still with the help of others, it seems that I really could be on the final stretch of this long journey. I only hope the sense of connection can last beyond my departure from the island, beyond my return to London, and to Max. I will need it for what comes next. I'll need people on hand when I stand still to let my thoughts of Granny near again. For the moment I stop running from what I've had, and what I've lost. At that point, more than ever, I'll need to keep that sense of connection alive.

Right now, at the buoy, there are no signs of sharks at the surface. With Libber standing at the helm, keeping a watchful gaze, the five of us get ready. We – *we* – will slip carefully into the water. We will not make a splash. We will look through our masks to see what we can.

I've no idea of the depth of the ocean below us, but I do know that there's no chance of seeing the bottom. That's OK – it's not scary right now – as long as I can look up and see the others. Simon and Chris. Rilke and Holly. Libber in the boat. We're all in this quest together. I plant my face back in the water. Blankness is all that's there, not even one visible speck of plankton, not one rolling wreath of weed.

After a minute, my mind veers to *Jaws*. The intermittent hum of a distant boat is hitting exactly the same notes as the soundtrack. Instinctively the tune begins to play inside my head.

'No,' I say. 'That's enough.' I breathe – in, out, in, out – and focus. And I get over it.

The others are roughly 15 metres away, clustered around the buoy itself, when I spot it: the dark silhouette of something huge with fins and a sweeping tail.

It cannot be, I think.

But it is.

'Shark,' I call, quietly, not wanting to disturb it. 'Whale shark,' I call again. I lift my head higher. Nobody has heard me. 'There's a whale shark,' I shout, more loudly. 'Over here!'

Rilke is the only one who picks up what I'm saying. Everyone else has their ears part-immersed in the ocean.

'Simon!' she calls. 'Chris! Georgie found one!'

Then Holly hears Rilke and joins in the game – keeps the relay going. 'Simon? Chris?'

I hear Simon say, 'Yep?'

'Georgie's got one.'

'You found a whale shark!' Simon yells.

'It's over here,' I say. My voice gets louder. 'About 10 metres down!'

Chris has heard now too. He hoots with pleasure. 'Well done, Georgie!'

I peer back into the water. It's still there, the whale shark, making its way through the current.

'Can you see it, Libber?' Chris calls to the boat.

'Yes!' Libber shouts.

'OK!'

We pile back onboard. We want to get closer. Libber will take us closer. From all around me come congratulations. It feels like I've earned my place on the boat. It feels like I've earned my place beside the whale shark. I am smiles and fidgeting. I am nervous excitement. Libber keeps an eye on the water. He gets us where we need to be, ahead of where the shark's going.

And then: 'Go in,' says Libber. 'Go now.'

When I slip into the water there it is. A male. An enormous male. So much closer than the others. So much bigger. So much – *there*.

'Eeee!' I cry. 'My God!'

My whale shark, our whale shark, swims about 2 metres, 3, below the surface, almost within touching distance of me. Its body is easily 8 metres long, maybe 9. Its head, its unfathomable head, looks purely Jurassic: wide and solid and ancient. Small remoras, suckerfish, are clustering under its belly, as if to protect themselves from the weight of the ocean; as if they have found an ally, and don't want to let go.

How something this large has come into existence, how something this large is swimming so gracefully now, how there are female whale sharks out there that are built to an added half this size again — all are enigmas I'll ponder hard in the weeks and months to come, unable to find any answers that work, apart from *That's just how it is*. Until then, this moment is happening and we're in it. Simon and Chris dive expertly deep with deft kicks of their fins, photographing the shark, observing, looking for signs of damage and old tracking tags. Rilke and Holly swim through the waves beside it, occasionally diving down for a closer look. A boat of tourists has seen our entry, and is preparing to shed its passengers alongside us. More boats will swiftly follow, we know. But there's still time to swim and marvel, to think of this shark as our own.

For one quick moment, while nobody else is down under, I feel an inexorable urge to leave the surface. I take a deep gulp of sea air and dive. I, diving. Just me. There I find not a fish in my reach but something more like a machine. The muscular ridges of its sides are like the contours of a military weapon. The girth and strength of its tail could knock down buildings. Its pectoral fins alone are human-sized. The size of it explodes my field of vision.

But the shark shows me no threat, nor any signs of being threatened.

Later, I will find out that our shark has a name. I will learn that he is called Rocky, and that he has coursed through these waters every year since he first was photographed, back in 2011. I will be asked if I want to change his name – they can do that, say Chris and Simon. But Rocky he is and Rocky he'll stay. Instead I'll be given the privilege of naming a nameless whale shark that we find an hour later, a shark that I'll circle with unrestrained awe and delight, that we'll keep to ourselves and will not have to share.

I will call that shark Buoy George. I will think about him and Rocky drifting through the currents. I will feel like invisible lines are linking us, as they link everyone who dwells in the sea.

But for the moment, swimming in the Indian Ocean, I can only gape at the strange way this shark, this Rocky, fills the space. Miraculously, it's not fearsome. Not with the sunshine dappling through the water. Not while he carries purposefully on, leisurely moving forward, permitting us to follow.

I'm forced to come out of the water seconds later. My lungs inhale a drag of salty air. Then I turn back down, kick hard with my fins, and the ocean swallows me up again. I'm metres from the whale shark, and his bulbous eye is suddenly, for the first time, looking back at me. Me and the shark in the water. Me and a shark, eye to eye. The whale shark looks away. What he thinks, if he thinks, is a mystery. What I think is that I have become a remora, taking temporary shelter, trying to make this indifferent creature my ally.

Ahead I can see that the shark's wide mouth is open, ever so slightly. I can see that his is not the mouth possessed by a Grim Reaper; a sucker of souls. Instead it is a curious mouth – a mouth seeking food, waiting for the northern winds to blow. I'm so close I can feel the current of his bulk pulling me in. I want this whale shark to carry me with it. Let him take me for a ride through this watery galaxy. But my lungs are about to run out of air once more.

I can see the legs of Rilke and Holly above me, Simon and Chris still at work. Then one small thought bubbles out of my wonder-filled brain: *I don't want this to end.*

The urge to breathe lifts me right back out again. Then the moment is over, passing me into the surging wave of the next one, and the next.

Author's Note

Even as I was catching my breath in Mafia, several things were shifting. They often do.

A few months after my final stint on the shop stool, James Deane sold his business to new owners. As I write this, he is still working there, part-time.

In spring 2019, the London Diving Chamber at St John's Wood (home to Vicky and crew) closed down having lost its funding after heavy NHS cuts. London Hyperbaric Medicine, at Whipps Cross Hospital, remains in operation, and now serves the entire London area.

Other details that I've covered here – not least the facts surrounding species lost and species found – are guaranteed to change. I hope that, one day, the better changes will overtake the worse ones.

References

Part One: We Swim

CHAPTER ONE: BIG FEAR

p. 9, Peter Benchley, 'Without malice: in defence of the shark', *G2 Magazine*, The *Guardian*, 9 November 2000

p. 9, Jacques-Yves Cousteau and Philippe Cousteau, *The Shark: Splendid Savage of the Sea*, translated by Francis Price. Arrowood Press, New York, 1987

p. 11, Jacques-Yves Cousteau and Philippe Diolé, *The Whale: Mighty Monarch of the Sea*, translated by J.F. Bernard. Arrowood Press, New York, 1972

CHAPTER TWO: STRANGE FISH

p. 29, Slaney Begley (editor), *Sharks*, Scholastic, New York, 2013

p. 30, Tyler Hart and Peter Buzzacott, 'Diver was virtually swallowed by whale shark', *Divers Alert Network*, www.diversalertnetwork.org/diving-incidents/ Diver-was-virtually-swallowed-by-a-whale-shark

p. 38, Celeste Brash, Austin Bush, David Eimer and Adam Skolnick, *Lonely Planet: Thailand's Islands and Beaches*, Lonely Planet Publications Pty Ltd, 2014

CHAPTER FIVE: DARK PLACES

p. 70, Margaret Codd, 'The Same Child from Eleven to Sixteen', published in *Recall: Anthology of Creative Writing by the*

Swindon Course, Newton Park College of Education, Pitman Press, Bath, 1966

p. 71, 'Drowning', *World Health Organization,* January 2018, www.who.int/news-room/fact-sheets/detail/drowning

p. 72, *Lonely Planet: Thailand's Islands and Beaches,* 2014

p. 84, Jacques-Yves Cousteau and Philippe Cousteau, *The Shark: Splendid Savage of the Sea*

CHAPTER SIX: DEEPER, DARKER

p. 88–9, John Bantin, *Amazing Diving Stories,* Fernhurst Books, Leamington Spa, 2014

p. 91, Tarek Omar interviewed by Maik Grossekathöfer, interviewed by Maik Grossekathöfer, 'The Bone Garden: A Visit to the World's Deadliest Dive Site', translated by Christopher Sultan, *Spiegel Online,* 13 July 2012, www. spiegel.de/international/zeitgeist/the-blue-hole-in-the-red-sea-is-the-deadliest-dive-site-in-the-world-a-844099-2.html

p. 91, Tarek Omar interviewed by Edmund Bower, 'Top diver's death casts long shadow over deep beauty of the Blue Hole', The *Observer,* 27 August 2017

p. 92, Tarek Omar interviewed by Niveen Ghoneim, 'Egyptian diver Tarek Omar: the keeper of Dahab's divers' cemetery', *Cairo Scene,* 20 October 2016, www.cairoscene.me/LifeStyle/ Egyptian-Diver-Tarek-Omar-The-Keeper-of-Dahab-s-Divers-Cemetery

CHAPTER SEVEN: TO RICHELIEU AND BEYOND

p. 103, Jacques-Yves Cousteau and Philippe Cousteau, *The Shark: Splendid Savage of the Sea*

CHAPTER EIGHT: A VOID

p. 118, Jacques-Yves Cousteau and Philippe Cousteau, *The Shark: Splendid Savage of the Sea*

p. 118, S.J. Pierce and B. Norman, 'Whale Shark, Rhincodon typus', *The IUCN Red List of Threatened Species,* 2016, www. iucnredlist.org/species/19488/2365291

p. 119, *Wildbook for Whale Sharks,* maintained and developed by Jason Holmberg, with oversight and guidance from Simon Pierce, www.whaleshark.org

p. 128, 'At Least 16 Die as Typhoon Sinks Barge Off Hong Kong', *Los Angeles Times*, 16 August 1991

p. 133, Sigmund Freud, *Beyond the Pleasure Principle*, translated by C.J.M. Hubback, The International Psychoanalytical Press, London, 1922

CHAPTER NINE: LEFT IN THE COLD

p. 139, Violet Jessop, *Titanic Survivor*, Sheridan House, New York, 1997

p. 139, Heikal Tawab interviewed in 'The Bone Garden: A Visit to the World's Deadliest Dive Site', *Spiegel Online*

Part Two: We Drift

p. 161, Margaret Codd, 'After Twenty Years', published in *Recall: Anthology of Creative Writing by the Swindon Course*

CHAPTER TEN: ONLY ONE WAY OUT

p. 168, Further details of Dean Upson's story can be found in his first-person account, '"I walked out covered in a young girl's blood": one soldier's struggle with PTSD, and the Ministry of Defence', The *Independent*, 22 August 2016

p. 174, Herman Melville, *Moby-Dick, or The Whale*, Wordsworth Editions Limited, Hertfordshire, 1993

CHAPTER ELEVEN: HERE BE MONSTERS

p. 191, Andrew Wight and John Garvin (writers), *Deepsea Challenge*, directed by John Bruno, Ray Quint and Andrew Wight, GEM Entertainment, 2014

p. 192, Douglas Adams, *The Restaurant at the End of the Universe*, Pan Books, London, 1980

p. 193, Herman Melville, *Moby-Dick, or The Whale*

p. 193, Jon Copley, 'No longer in the dark – the future of the deep oceans', *TEDx Southampton University*, published online by TEDx Talks, 13 May 2013, www.tedxsouthamptonuniversity. wordpress.com/the-2013-event

p. 196, press release, 'Over 1,000 New Ocean Fish Species Identified In Past Eight Years, Including 122 Sharks, Rays', *LifeWatch* and the *World Register of Marine Species*, 12 March 2015, www. lifewatch.be/en/2015.03.12-WoRMS-LifeWatch-press-release

p. 197, National Ocean Service, 'How much of the ocean have we explored?' *National Oceanic and Atmospheric Administration*, U.S. Department of Commerce, 11 July 2018, www. oceanservice.noaa.gov/facts/exploration.html

CHAPTER FOURTEEN: OPEN-MOUTHED

p. 237, Alex Wright, *The Dream of Hieronymus Sloth*, Delderfield Press Limited, Exmouth, 1973

CHAPTER FIFTEEN: NORTHWEST PASSAGE

p. 263, Tex Geddes, *Hebridean Sharker*, Birlinn Limited, Edinburgh, 2012

p. 266, Gavin Naylor and Tyler Bowling, '2017 Yearly Worldwide Shark Attack Summary', *International Shark Attack File*, University of Florida, 2018, www.floridamuseum.ufl.edu/ shark-attacks/yearly-worldwide-summary

p. 268, Thor Heyerdahl, *Kon-Tiki: Across the Pacific by Raft*, translated by F.H. Lyon, Simon & Schuster, London, 1973

Further Reading and Resources

I recommend the following material for readers wanting more background on the themes and topics covered in this book.

BOOKS

Victoria Braithwaite, *Do Fish Feel Pain?* Oxford University Press, Oxford, 2010
> A carefully objective study on the facts surrounding fish and their pain responses. Thought-provoking and readable.

Jacques-Yves Cousteau, *The Ocean World*, Abradale Press and Harry N. Abrams Inc., New York, 1985
> An enormous collection of sea-themed essays on topics including Cousteau's attempts to establish underwater colonies with his crew.

Jacques-Yves Cousteau with Frederic Dumas, *The Silent World*, Hamish Hamilton Limited, London, 1952
> The original scuba book by the father of diving. Features the unforgettable lines: 'For reasons of their own, women are suspicious of diving and frown on their menfolk going down. Dumas, who has starred in seven underwater films, has never received a fan letter from a woman.'

Oliver Firth and Jules Eden, *FAQ Dive Medicine,* Quetzal
Publishing, London, 2012
> An entertaining compendium of dive-themed medical
> questions, complete with informative answers.

Lee Griffiths, *A Simple Guide to Decompression Illness*, AquaPress,
Southend-on-Sea, 2010
> A compact, detailed and knowledgeable guide written
> by a hyperbaric specialist, formerly of Whipps Cross
> Hospital, London.

FILM

Jacques-Yves Cousteau (writer), *The Silent World*, directed
by Jacques-Yves Cousteau and Louis Malle, Columbia
Pictures, 1956
> A colourful documentary that inspired a generation of scuba
> divers. Its occasional use of harpoons and explosives may
> disturb contemporary viewers.

Alex Parkinson (writer), *Last Breath*, directed by Alex Parkinson
and Richard da Costa, BBC, 2018
> A suspenseful docu-drama that tells the story of Chris
> Lemons, a saturation diver stranded on the floor of the
> North Sea, with only five minutes of oxygen in his tank. A
> window onto modern sat diving practices.

Juan Reina (writer), *Diving Into The Unknown*, directed by Juan
Reina, B-Plan Distribution, 2016
> A dramatic account of a real-life diving disaster and its
> consequences, occurring deep within a Norwegian cave
> system. Provides a rich insight into mindsets involved in
> cave-diving.

ONLINE COURSE

Sharks! Global Biodiversity, Biology and Conservation, created by
The University of Queensland and Cornell University, 2016
> A free and comprehensive introduction to shark studies,
> featuring videos, quizzes and more. Recommended by

a number of marine biologists. www.edx.org/course/
sharks-global-biodiversity-biology-cornellx-uqx-bioee101x

RADIO

Julia DeWitt (producer), *Where No One Should Go*, Snap
Judgment Studios, WNYC, Oakland, 2014
> The true tale of deep-diver Dave Shaw and his courageous
> mission to recover the body of Deon Dreyer from Bushman's
> Hole, South Africa.

WEBSITES

For the watery things in life

Georgia Aquarium, www.georgiaaquarium.org
> Atlanta-based aquarium with a friendly research and
> conservation team.

Help for Heroes, www.helpforheroes.org.uk
> Charity for British ex-servicemen, and women, with
> injuries/illnesses attributable to their time in the Armed
> Forces. Runs diver training in its Sports Recovery scheme.

Large Marine Vertebrates Research Institute Philippines,
www.lamave.org
> Non-government organisation dedicated to ocean
> conservation, with an extensive cache of freely accessible
> papers. Hosts a range of volunteer placements.

Marine Megafauna Foundation,
www.marinemegafaunafoundation.org
> Global charity aiming to develop lasting, positive strategies
> that will benefit marine megafauna. Publishes research and
> leads worldwide expeditions to raise funds.

National Oceanic and Atmospheric Association,
www.noaa.gov
> American agency working to research, understand and
> predict environmental change for the protection and
> conservation of marine ecosystems.

Professional Association of Diving Instructors, www.padi.com
    International dive training body, certifying more than 27
    million students in 53 years.

Whale Shark and Oceanic Research Centre, www.wsorc.org
    Honduras-based not-for-profit that has been gathering data
    on whale sharks since 1997. Runs internships and research
    opportunities.

Wildbook for Whale Sharks, www.whaleshark.org
    Go-to site for all registered whale shark sightings, using
    NASA-inspired photo-identification technology.

World Register of Marine Species, www.marinespecies.org
    Continually updated database containing names of all
    known marine organisms. Its press releases on new
    discoveries attract global media attention.

And for life in general

Mind, the Mental Health Charity, www.mind.org.uk
    A hub for anyone seeking help for mental health issues,
    including anxiety, bereavement and depression.

Sapper Support, www.sappersupport.com
    Listening and support charity for PTSD sufferers, staffed by
    UK veterans and 999 personnel. Runs a free 24/7 helpline
    and can fund PTSD assessments.

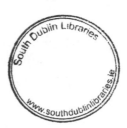

Acknowledgements

It can take a lot of people to find a shark – and even more to write about it.

I'd like to thank the story sharers, brilliant friends, and adventurous contacts I've made over the course of this book, from 2015 to 2019, especially those who brightened (and, in some cases, set in motion) my journeys through Thailand, Mexico, Scotland and Tanzania. They include, but are not limited to, Adam D., Ahmed G., Alex G., Andrew K., Bruce C., Bryony H., Carly P., Chris R., Clare F., Dan H., David R., Dean U., Emma L., Holly, James D., Jamie H., Jason H., Jen K., John G., Jon C., Laura L., Libber M., Liv P., Mungo W., Paige H., Paul C., Rilke, Rob J., Sally S., Simon P., Tarek O., Vas P., Vicky B. and Wayne F.

Rent and food costs for part of my writing period were funded by the Society of Authors, for which I'm extremely grateful. My gratitude for what remains of the British library system is also huge. Like lots of readers I hope to see it restored to its former glory one day.

Huge thanks to my agent Ed Wilson, and my editor Rhiannon Smith, plus Meryl, Nithya and Sophie from Fleet, for their excitement, humour and first-rate attention to detail.

Huge thanks to my excellent friends in London, Norwich

and beyond, many of whom were encouraging readers (and ultra-helpful critics). Alex, Bridie, Ellie, Jez, Mandi, Saf, Tom B. – this includes you.

Huge thanks to my family for their enthusiasm, and to my mother especially, for all of her hard graft, not to mention her unfailing support for my work.

Thank you, Max, for constantly finding ways to make me smile.

And thank you, Granny, for enriching my life with cooking, word games and weekly trips to the library. This book could not have existed without you and Mum. Neither could I, come to think of it.